Rightsizing

APPROPRIATE STAFFING FOR YOUR MEDICAL PRACTICE

Deborah L. Walker, MBA, FACMPE

David N. Gans, MSHA, CMPE

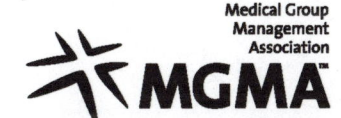

Medical Group Management Association
104 Inverness Terrace East
Englewood, CO 80112
877.275.6462
Web site: www.mgma.com

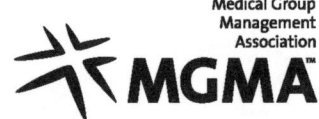

Medical Group Management Association (MGMA) publications are intended to provide current and accurate information and are designed to assist readers in becoming more familiar with the subject matter covered. Such publications are distributed with the understanding that MGMA does not render any legal, accounting or other professional advice that may be construed as specifically applicable to individual situations. No representations or warranties are made concerning the application of legal or other principles discussed by the authors to any specific factual situation, nor is any prediction made concerning how any particular judge, government official or other person will interpret or apply such principles. Specific factual situations should be discussed with professional advisors.

Cover photo courtesy of PhotoDisc, Inc.

Item # 5692

Copyright © 2003 by Deborah L. Walker, MBA, FACMPE and the Medical Group Management Association

ISBN 1-56829-149-3

All rights reserved. No part of this publication may be reproduced, stored in a retrieval system, or transmitted, in any form or by any means, electronic, mechanical, photocopying, recording, or otherwise, without the prior written permission of the copyright owner.

Printed in the United States of America
10 9 8 7 6 5 4 3 2

Dedication

*This book is dedicated to our parents,
Wilma and George Boehm and Hope and Harry Gans, who
instilled a love of learning,
and to our spouses,
Mike Keegan and Joan Gans,
who encourage us to pursue our dreams.*

Contents

CHAPTER 1 ■ What Is Rightsizing? 1

    Definition of Rightsizing   **1**
    Myths About Rightsizing   **2**

CHAPTER 2 ■ Why Rightsize the Medical Practice? 5

    Management of the Knowledge Worker   **5**
    Current Labor Market   **6**
    Four Generations at Work   **6**
    Employees As Resources, Not Simply Costs   **7**
    Consequences of "Wrongsizing"   **7**

CHAPTER 3 ■ How Staffing Levels Affect Medical Practice Profitability 11

    Rightsizing   **11**
    What You Cannot Measure, You Cannot Manage   **12**
    How Do Practices Staff?   **12**
    Understanding Constraints   **13**
    Increased Profitability Is Associated with Rightsized Staffing   **26**
    Applying General Performance Information to a Specific Practice   **27**

CHAPTER 4 ■ Staffing Is a Measure of Work 29

    Linking Staff to Physician Work Levels   **29**
    Impact of Medical or Surgical Specialty on Staffing   **29**
    Impact of Physician Productivity and Practice Scope on Staffing   **30**

CHAPTER 5 ■ The Impact of Internal Practice-Specific Factors on Rightsizing 35

    Practice Model   **35**
    Patient Scheduling   **40**
    Practice Facility   **41**
    Technology   **42**

CHAPTER 6 ■ A Systematic Approach to Rightsizing the Medical Practice 45

    Step 1: Benchmark the Current State   **47**
    Step 2: Analyze Current Productivity   **64**
    Step 3: Analyze the Current Practice Model   **67**
    Step 4: Analyze Process Performance   **68**
    Step 5: Take Action   **73**

CHAPTER 7 ■ A Closer Look at Staffing Categories and Staffing Models 75

General Administrative Staff **75**
Billing Office Staff **76**
Front Office Staff **78**
Medical Records Staff **79**
Clinical Support Staff **80**
Ancillary Staff **81**
Outsourcing Job Functions **83**
Staffing for Seasonality **84**

Conclusion and Future Implications 87

Appendixes 89

I. Frequently Asked Questions **91**
II. Staffing Resource Allocation Tool **93**
III. MGMA Benchmarks—Peer Comparison Tables **105**
IV. MGMA Benchmarks—Better Performing Practices Comparison Tables **165**
V. MGMA Definitions of Support Staff Positions **177**

Acknowledgments

We are grateful to Sara Larch, MS, FACMPE, and Elizabeth Woodcock, MBA, FACMPE for their insights and expertise and for providing critical comment on an earlier draft of this manuscript. We also wish to thank Kristin Russell, Mary Mourar and Bob Redling of the Medical Group Management Association for their valuable input and support of this project.

About the Authors

Deborah L. Walker, MBA, FACMPE, is a principal with BOEHM/WALKER Associates. She assists medical practices and health care organizations in reducing administrative costs, improving productivity and efficiency and developing physician compensation systems. With over 22 years of experience in health care, including serving as a health care administrator for the University of California system and as a health care consultant, Ms. Walker has developed a special expertise in implementing organizational changes and productivity improvement to enable a competitive position in managed care markets. Ms. Walker is a Phi Beta Kappa graduate of UCLA, and she received her MBA from UCLA's Anderson Graduate School of Business. She is a Fellow of the American College of Medical Practice Executives, and she is currently a PhD Candidate at the Peter F. Drucker Graduate School of Management, Claremont Graduate University. Her dissertation is entitled "Management Coordination Systems in Health System Networks." Ms. Walker has authored numerous articles on medical practice operations issues, and she is a frequent keynote speaker at national health care forums.

David N. Gans, CMPE, is Director of Practice Management Resources for the Medical Group Management Association (MGMA) in Englewood, Colorado, where he is the MGMA staff expert on medical group practice management. He is an educational program speaker, author of a monthly column in *MGMA Connexion,*™ and he provides technical assistance to the association's staff and members on the topic areas of benchmarking, use of survey data, financial management, cost efficiency, physician compensation and productivity, managerial compensation, the Resource Based Relative Value Scale (RBRVS), employee staffing, cost accounting, medical group organization and emergency preparedness. He is a retired Colonel in the United States Army Reserve. Mr. Gans earned an undergraduate degree in government at the University of Notre Dame, a master's degree in education from the University of Southern California, and a master of science degree in health administration from the University of Colorado. He is a certified member of the American College of Medical Practice Executives.

The idea for this book originated from a national MGMA audio conference conducted by the authors on this topic. The examples used in this publication were developed to illustrate staff rightsizing concepts and tools and do not reflect actual medical practices.

Deborah L. Walker	David N. Gans
BOEHM/Walker Associates	Medical Group Management Association
Surfside, California	Englewood, Colorado

Introduction

What Is Our Goal?
The right number of staff, in the right place, with the right skills,
at the right cost, with the right behavior, with the right rewards,
with the right outcomes—no more, no less.

Rightsizing staff in the medical practice is important not only to ensure optimal physician productivity, but also to ensure practice profitability and performance. Better performing practices—those practices that stand-out from their peers on critical quantitative dimensions—take a specific, systematic approach to rightsizing their staff. They take steps to ensure that the practice makes optimal use of its resources and infrastructure to support physician productivity. Each medical practice is unique; however, a systematic approach toward rightsizing will permit practices to discover their opportunities to rightsize staff and to enhance the critical business processes that promote efficient and effective performance.

This book outlines a systematic approach to rightsizing staff. It provides the tools and techniques that medical groups need to ensure that they have the right number of staff, doing the right things, with the right resources to ensure optimal physician productivity, practice efficiency, profitability and performance.

This book is organized along the following chapter lines:

CHAPTER 1: WHAT IS RIGHTSIZING?

This chapter provides a definition of rightsizing the medical practice. Four common myths are dispelled related to staff rightsizing.

CHAPTER 2: WHY RIGHTSIZE THE MEDICAL PRACTICE?

The business risk of having either too many staff or too few staff is described. In this chapter, readers will learn the importance of conducting a systematic rightsizing process.

CHAPTER 3: HOW STAFFING LEVELS AFFECT MEDICAL PRACTICE PROFITABILITY

MGMA survey data suggest an association between increased profitability and rightsized staffing. This chapter discusses the impact of staff rightsizing on practice profitability as measured by revenue after operating expenses per FTE physician. At the lowest and often at the highest levels of staffing, practices report lower levels of financial performance, suggesting the importance of staff rightsizing to the profitability of the medical practice.

CHAPTER 4: STAFFING IS A MEASURE OF WORK

The concept of "staffing is a measure of work" is detailed in this chapter. Staffing levels within a practice will vary based upon physician productivity, scope of services provided acuity of services provided and practice specialty. Data from MGMA survey instruments are provided to support this concept.

CHAPTER 5: THE IMPACT OF INTERNAL PRACTICE-SPECIFIC FACTORS ON RIGHTSIZING

The impacts of four key internal medical practice-specific factors on staff rightsizing are explored. The four factors include 1) the practice model that has been adopted, 2) the patient scheduling methods, 3) the size and layout of the practice's facility, and 4) the practice's use of technology.

CHAPTER 6: A SYSTEMATIC APPROACH TO RIGHTSIZING THE MEDICAL PRACTICE

This chapter describes a five-step process to rightsize staff in the medical practice:

Step 1: Benchmark the Current State
Step 2: Analyze Current Productivity
Step 3: Analyze the Current Practice Model
Step 4: Analyze Work Processes
Step 5: Take Action

A case study approach is used to demonstrate Step 1—Benchmark the Current State, and situations specific to medical practice are provided to demonstrate Steps 2, 3 and 4 of the rightsizing process.

CHAPTER 7: A CLOSER LOOK AT STAFFING CATEGORIES AND STAFFING MODELS

This chapter takes a detailed look at specific staffing categories, including general administrative staff, billing office staff, front office staff, medical records staff, clinical support staff and ancillary staff. The concept of building staff levels based on job functions is advanced. Outsourcing specific medical practice functions and adopting a different staffing model during fluctuating patient demand are also explored.

CONCLUSION AND FUTURE IMPLICATIONS

Future implications of rightsizing staff and the need to continuously review staffing models, staffing levels and staffing workload are emphasized. In addition, the importance of effective human resource management processes for staff rightsizing, including articulating performance expectations, conducting performance management processes and balancing formal and informal rewards is noted in order to recruit, develop and retain a high performing support staff.

APPENDIXES

Appendix I: Frequently Asked Questions

Answers to frequently asked questions regarding the staff rightsizing process are provided in Appendix I.

Appendix II: Staffing Resource Allocation Tool

A tool to assist in the staff rightsizing process is provided in Appendix II. This tool incorporates both quantitative and qualitative measures to review a particular staff position in the medical practice for rightsizing opportunity.

Appendix III: MGMA Benchmarks—Peer Comparison Tables

This Appendix provides the key staffing benchmarks to be used in Step 1—Benchmark the Current State when comparing a practice's staffing to those of its **peers.** The data include benchmarks at the **staff category level** (administrative and business staff, front office staff, clinical staff, and ancillary service staff) as well as the **staff job classification level** for 28 different specialties and group practice ownership categories.

Appendix IV: MGMA Benchmarks—Better Performing Practices Comparison Tables

Appendix IV provides the key staffing benchmarks to be used in Step 1—Benchmark the Current State, when comparing a practice's staffing to those of **better performing medical practices.** The data include benchmarks at the **staff category level** (administrative and business staff, front office staff, clinical staff and ancillary service staff), as well as at the **staff job classification level** for five different medical practice types: multispecialty groups, cardiology, family practice, obstetrics & gynecology and orthopedic surgery.

Appendix V: MGMA Definitions of Support Staff Positions

This Appendix contains definitions of the support staff categories and the specific job classifications within each category in order to facilitate benchmarking comparison to the MGMA data. The job classifications are grouped into four distinct staff categories: administrative and business staff, front office staff, clinical staff and ancillary service staff.

CHAPTER 1

What Is Rightsizing?

■ DEFINITION OF RIGHTSIZING

Rightsizing is the systematic review of staffing levels, tasks and work processes to determine the appropriate number and mix of staff needed to meet medical practice goals. Rightsizing is practice-specific. It is influenced by physician expectations, physician productivity and internal practice-specific limiting factors such as a practice's facility and technology. The specific actions that will accomplish rightsizing will vary based upon the internal limiting factors of the medical practice, as well as its group culture and strategic and operational goals. Rightsizing does not involve embracing arbitrary targets or goals. Rather, it is a systematic approach to staffing work conducted in the medical practice.

The Medical Group Management Association (MGMA) data associated with staffing deployment in the medical group present a clear picture of the importance of rightsizing the medical practice. **According to the MGMA data, at the lowest and often at the highest levels of staffing, medical practices report lower levels of financial performance.**

Low staffing levels constrain physician productivity. Physicians in under-staffed practices may be more involved in non-clinical, administrative tasks and may lack the necessary infrastructure to support their clinical productivity and efficiency, as well as the practice's profitability. In addition, low staffing levels can present a business risk to a medical group if they introduce greater variability in work processes and performance, lead to problematic patient access and service, and create poor staff morale that results in high staff turnover.

At the highest levels of staffing, the data show that the increased cost of staff does not translate to higher performance as measured by revenue after operating cost. Better performing medical groups are those that have identified the best number and best mix of staff

FIGURE 1.1 ■ Definition of Rightsizing

> Rightsizing is the systematic process of reviewing staffing levels, tasks and work processes to determine the appropriate number and mix of staff needed to meet medical practice goals.

to support physician productivity and make a positive financial impact on the medical group.

The authors firmly believe that employees in the medical practice are the practice's most valuable resource. They have witnessed firsthand the effects on both the practice and its employees when the staff is "wrongsized" versus "rightsized." They have also witnessed the role of employees in a practice's ultimate success. It still matters how the telephone scheduler interacts with the patient to promote ease of access to the practice. It still matters if patients are greeted and warmly welcomed to the practice, or if they are treated like a number or like a disease. It still matters that the nurse reflects empathy and concern and assists the physician in caring for the patient as a human being, not just as a customer.

It is important to note that some researchers have identified a "mirror" phenomenon associated with employee satisfaction and customer satisfaction.[1] That is, when high levels of employee satisfaction are reported, high levels of customer satisfaction are also found. This "mirror" test holds true in the medical practice. Rightsizing makes a tremendous impact on employee satisfaction. Employees who feel frenzied or too hurried in their job assignments rarely report high job satisfaction. However, it is equally important to recognize that rightsizing staff has implications for patient satisfaction, a critical performance measure of medical practices today.

MYTHS ABOUT RIGHTSIZING

There are a number of myths about rightsizing that we want to dispel early on. Rightsizing is not a panacea to resolve problematic productivity and profitability issues for a medical practice. Rather, it is a systematic approach to ensure that the practice has sufficient and appropriate human resources to achieve optimal performance levels.

MYTH #1: RIGHTSIZING ALWAYS MEANS DOWNSIZING

Rightsizing does not mean layoffs. Rightsizing may mean that *more* staff is needed or a different skill mix of staff is needed in order to meet the practice's goals and objectives. Thus, rightsizing will not necessarily lead to downsizing. High numbers of layoffs often indicate that the medical practice has not systematically rightsized—that is, it has not continuously assessed whether staffing volume, skill mix and workload are consistent with its current state and future goals.

FIGURE 1.2 ■ Myths about Rightsizing

1. Rightsizing always means downsizing
2. Rightsizing translates to cost savings
3. Rightsizing decreases physician productivity
4. Rightsizing results in decreased patient satisfaction

---

[1] Heskett JL, Sasser WE, Schlesinger LA. The Service Profit Chain. New York: The Free Press; 1997.

MYTH #2: RIGHTSIZING TRANSLATES TO COST SAVINGS

Rightsizing staff does not necessarily translate to cost savings for the medical practice. The practice may need more staff or a different skill mix of staff that may lead to higher staffing costs. The practice may need to use technology or make a significant change to process performance in order to increase productivity or efficiency that may lead to higher general operating costs. Although rightsizing may reduce staffing cost as a percent of total medical revenue, this outcome is not assured.

MYTH #3: RIGHTSIZING DECREASES PHYSICIAN PRODUCTIVITY

If, after a practice rightsizes its staff, physician productivity decreases, then the practice has not rightsized; it has definitely "wrongsized." The medical practice's personnel are the infrastructure and resources necessary to support physician productivity. If, as a result of rightsizing, physicians spend more time in non-clinical, administrative tasks, then rightsizing has not been achieved. Regardless of whether or not the medical practice is situated in a highly managed care environment, most physicians must see large panels of patients for the practice to remain financially viable. Rightsizing should promote, rather than thwart physician productivity.

MYTH #4: RIGHTSIZING RESULTS IN DECREASED PATIENT SERVICE

The last myth we wish to dispel is one that suggests that changes to staffing volumes and skill mix of staff result in reduced patient service. The service delivery challenge in healthcare is not non-trivial. In fact, many patients view service as a proxy for healthcare quality. If, after rightsizing its staff, the medical practice's patient satisfaction scores decline, the practice must immediately investigate the root cause of this decline. If a critical function or role changed as a result of rightsizing and it impacts patient perceptions of service, then intervention is necessary to resolve this dilemma. We do not advocate rightsizing that decreases patient access, service or patient satisfaction.

CHAPTER 2

Why Rightsize the Medical Practice?

The following current trends in human resources management provide strong support for rightsizing staff in the medical practice:

1. Medical practice management involves managing knowledge workers;
2. The current labor market limits the practice's ability to recruit qualified staff;
3. There are now four generations at work in medical practices; and
4. Employees are the infrastructure and support for physician productivity, not simply a cost of doing business.

■ 1. MANAGEMENT OF THE KNOWLEDGE WORKER

Healthcare is not your typical commodity. The skill, talent, and experience of physicians and staff are vital to ensure quality clinical care. These individuals are indeed "knowledge workers" in every sense of the term. Peter Drucker notes that a key management challenge for the 21st century is to manage productivity of the knowledge worker, those individuals who possess intellectual capital required to perform their job.[2]

The staff in a medical practice is composed of knowledge workers. These employees possess the knowledge or intellectual capital that the practice needs to schedule appointments, treat patients, verify insurance, obtain pre-authorizations, code billable services, perform payment posting and adjustments, and perform insurance follow-up, among other tasks. Rare is the medical practice in which the exact approach to completing these various tasks is written down. The knowledge that employees need to perform their jobs is in their heads, and it is highly portable. Medical groups can ill afford to lose this vital practice resource to competitors. Rightsizing staff can ensure that the employees have acceptable workloads, that the practice has the right number of staff to ensure effective service and quality patient care, and that employees apply their considerable knowledge to further the organization's goals.

---

[2] Drucker PF. Management Challenges for the 21st Century. New York: Harper Business; 1999.

2. CURRENT LABOR MARKET

Despite a current tight labor market, there is still a shortage of skilled workers in the health care service industry. In many markets it is difficult to recruit individuals who are trained in front office medical practice operations or in physician professional fee billing. A nursing shortage has also contributed to difficulty in recruiting and retaining qualified nursing staff for ambulatory practice. Ensuring that the staff is rightsized can help the practice recognize the work level and scope of activity that staff should perform. It can prevent the tendency to simply add layer upon layer of initiatives to an already high workload.

In order to recruit and retain qualified administrative, business, front office, clinical and ancillary support staff, many practices offer innovative compensation and benefit plans. These include memberships to health clubs, payment of college tuition for immediate family members, veterinary benefits for employees' pets and even a two-week all-expense paid vacation (after 10 years of employment). A plastic surgery practice offers staff a free aesthetic procedure (up to $5,000). A dermatology practice offers staff free skin treatments. Another practice provides free lunches daily. Many practices have developed incentive plans that provide employees a share of practice profitability or bonus payments based upon group or team performance.

Other practices are working hard to emphasize the intangible benefits of working in a medical practice. They focus on building a "recognition culture" within the organization.[3] They do this by involving staff in decision-making, developing informal rewards and expanding the breadth and scope of responsibility for staff, among other activities.

Finally, researchers are revisiting the cost of staff turnover. Once it was assumed that replacing a staff member costs the practice 200 percent of the person's annual salary. Recent studies attempt to document such costs as the loss of intellectual capital, the impact on morale of employees who remain in the practice, the impact on patient satisfaction and other "opportunity costs." Thus, the cost of staff turnover will likely increase in the future.[4]

3. FOUR GENERATIONS AT WORK

Many researchers point to the challenge of managing a workforce that is cross-generational.[5] For the first time, there are four separate generations in the workplace. Each generation brings different values to the job.

While the authors are reluctant to classify individuals into distinct categories, there does seem to be some validity to discussions of generational differences in the workplace. Many managers say that it seems harder to manage employees today than in the past.

Using the terms set out by Zemke, et al, and other authors, some employees in the medical practice can be categorized as "Veterans," those individuals born between 1922 and 1943 who believe in sacrifice, honor, duty, and rules. In today's workplace there is a host of "Baby Boomers" (born between 1943 and 1960) who believe in work and involvement, personal growth and work teams, with a focus on health and maintenance of their youth. The "Gen-

---

[3] Nelson, B. Dissertation Presentation, Claremont University, April 21, 2001.
[4] Employee retention: What managers can do. Harvard Management Update, April 2001; 5(4).
[5] Zemke R, Raines C, Filipczak B. Generations at Work: Managing the Class of Veterans, Boomers, Xers, and Nexters in Your Workplace. New York: American Management Association (AMACOM), 1999.

Xers" in the workplace (born between 1960 and 1980) are those techno-literate and self-reliant staff who seek a balance between their professional and personal lives. And finally, some of our newest staff members are "Nexters." These are the individuals born between 1980 and the year 2000. Although we are not certain of their final disposition, we do know that they appear to have high confidence in themselves and they value individualism and diversity.[6] For most industries the management of four generations at work presents significant challenges. In the healthcare industry, one of the most complex industries within which to work, the challenge of managing and rightsizing a multigenerational staff is staggering.

4. EMPLOYEES AS RESOURCES, NOT SIMPLY COSTS

A final compelling argument for rightsizing staff relates to a common misperception that equates staff with "costs," rather than recognizes staff as resources.[7] While support staff salary and benefit costs are a significant practice expense, the classic scenario of reducing staff when revenue falls short of expectations is short-sighted, and often does not represent a sound business approach.

When there is a revenue shortfall, the first response of many medical practices is to cut supply expenditures, place educational opportunities on hold, or attempt to cut staff by 5 to 10 percent. This scenario may have a short-term financial benefit; however, it may also lead to a substantial increase in business risk for the medical practice. If the practice was already rightsized, a reduction in staff may lead to:

1. high process variability;
2. physicians performing administrative, non-clinical tasks; and/or
3. staff performing "out of class" assignments (for example, medical assistants performing licensed practical nurse functions which could increase patient safety risk or nursing staff performing basic clerical tasks).

This approach also treats employees as if they are merely costs in the medical practice, rather than recognizing that support staff in a medical practice are knowledge workers who provide the infrastructure and resources to support physician productivity and quality care. The consequences of this business risk for the medical practice make a compelling argument for rightsizing to ensure appropriate staffing levels, skill mix, staff assignment and workload in the medical practice.

CONSEQUENCES OF "WRONGSIZING"

In light of the above staffing challenges—management of the knowledge worker, a tight labor market, four generations at work and a tendency to view employees as costs—it is imperative that rightsizing be conducted with due diligence. A medical practice that is inadvertently "wrongsized" faces significant consequences. The complex and dynamic health care environment requires that medical practices generally get it right the first time when

---

[6]Ibid.

[7]Mozena JP, Emerick CE, Black SC. Stop Managing Costs: Designing Healthcare Organizations around Core Business Systems. Milwaukee: ASQ Quality Press; 1999.

FIGURE 2.1 ■ Consequences of Wrongsizing

Too Few Staff:
- Negative impact to staff recruitment and retention
- Physician productivity
- Problematic patient service
- Increased business risk
- Increased patient safety risk

Too Many Staff:
- Low staff productivity levels
- Negative financial impacts to the medical practice
- Inability to link staff with physician work levels

staffing the medical practice. There are few second chances once loss of patient service, financial losses, or other negative consequences of wrongsizing occur.

TOO FEW STAFF

The consequences of two few staff are many. Staff recruitment and retention are difficult for practices with too few staff. Employees are highly mobile, and they can seek alternative employment with practices that have appropriate staffing and workload levels.

Physician productivity will also decline with too few staff, because physicians will spend significant time on non-clinical, administrative tasks instead of providing health care services. Most practices can ill afford for their physicians to not be actively engaged in the clinical practice of medicine.

Too few staff also can lead to problematic patient service. Asking staff to handle more than an appropriate work level or scope of work will negatively impact patient service (and possibly patient safety). Staff cannot be "customer-minded" when they are racing through the day attempting to meet unrealistic workload demands.

A practice may also increase its business risk when it has an insufficient number of staff or an inappropriate skill mix of staff. Examples of the risk a practice faces when it has too few staff include: declines in the quality of patient care services, failure to appropriately manage the acuity level of patients, and overlooking important details. Also, when employees are asked to perform their tasks too quickly, internal controls may be de-emphasized and there is a tendency to cut corners. Medical practices with too few staff often resort to high levels of multi-tasking that typically result in low levels of accountability, since no one person can be held accountable for performance results. Thus, too few staff may lead to preventable business risk. It also may lead to expensive human resource issues such as excessive sick leave, labor issues or lawsuits because staff is required to perform workload levels or skill levels well beyond their current capability or training.

TOO MANY STAFF

The consequences of too many staff are also significant. A key question that should be asked is: *Do the staff act to influence physician productivity, or are they occupied with tasks that do not add value for the patient?* Staffing is a measure of work, thus the staffing levels would be expected to vary based upon medical and surgical procedures performed in the practice, work relative value units and other measures of physician work levels.

When there is an over-capacity of staff, employees become accustomed to low workload levels. This makes it very difficult to step up to higher levels of productivity. Many practices have too many staff because their staffing plan is based on meeting the maximum expected patient load at all times, when, in fact, patient volume fluctuates. (Chapter 7 discusses practice model options to meet fluctuating patient demand.)

There is obviously a financial impact associated with too many staff as well. Support staff expenditures as a percent of total medical revenue are high for those practices with too many staff. Staffing cost is one of the highest expenditures in the medical practice, typically ranging from 12 percent of total medical revenue for cardiovascular surgery to 32 percent for family practice, so actively managing staffing cost levels is important for practice profitability.

The practice's inability to adjust staff levels with the workload in the practice also represents a high cost staffing model. Some practices do not fluctuate their staffing consistent with physician schedules and the actual workload. For example, if surgeons are in the operating room on Tuesdays and Thursdays, then why does the practice need all of its staff in the office setting on those days? If Friday afternoons are lightly scheduled, why isn't staffing flexed to correspond with the lightened workload? Practices may argue that employees need this time to "catch up." However, medical practices today do not typically have the financial luxury of providing "catch up" time for staff when the physician is not scheduled. A final example of failure to match staffing with physician workload are those practices where physicians may work a four or four and one-half day workweek in the office, and the clinical support staff is flexed off with their physician, yet the staff still reports full-time hours due to overtime incurred during the workweek. This scenario does not permit the medical practice to take advantage of fluctuating work schedules and financial savings consistent with physician work levels.

In summary, there are significant costs to a medical practice if it has too few or too many support staff. It is critical to rightsize staff with the appropriate methodology and tools to perform this analysis correctly on the first attempt. Then, the practice must systematically rightsize its staff over time.

CHAPTER 3

How Staffing Levels Affect Medical Practice Profitability

Authors' Note: Portions of this chapter appeared in the MGMA "Performance and Practices of Successful Medical Groups: 2001 Report Based on 2000 Data." We thank MGMA for permission to publish this revised version.

■ RIGHTSIZING

In the best possible case, a medical practice will have the right number of staff, doing the right things, with the right resources, with the right outcomes, attaining optimal physician productivity to achieve maximum practice profitability.

Unfortunately, this situation exists only in theory. In reality, medical groups have different levels of staffing, doing both the right, and occasionally, the wrong things, with varying resources, achieving different levels of physician productivity and very different financial results. Only by examining the actual performance of many different practices can one understand what is the right size for a medical practice's support staff.

Staffing is only one factor that determines overall performance. It is heavily influenced by many other factors as well, including: physician practice style, group culture, operational goals, competitive market factors and internal practice-specific limiting factors, such as the size and layout of the practice's facility and its use of technology.

In order to understand the rightsize for its staff, a practice must first understand the objectives it wants to achieve. A practice can have numerous objectives, some of which can be contradictory, while others are complimentary. Examples of practice objectives include:

- Optimizing quality of care;
- Optimizing patient satisfaction;
- Minimizing medical errors;
- Optimizing practice revenue;
- Maximizing physician compensation; and
- Lessening the provider workweek.

Some of these objectives are easily quantifiable, others less so, and still others cannot be quantified at all.

■ WHAT YOU CANNOT MEASURE, YOU CANNOT MANAGE

In order to understand the effect of staffing on practice performance, performance measures must be selected that closely define what is meant by "success." Ideally, the performance measures should be directly related to the practice's strategic plan and business goals and objectives. However, it is imperative that the performance measures be quantifiable with a consistent scale, so that changes can be monitored to evaluate performance at various staffing levels.

For medical group practices, the best single measure of financial success is revenue after operating cost. This metric is calculated by subtracting total operating expenses from total medical revenue. In a medical group legally organized as a partnership or professional corporation, this value is typically the amount available to compensate the practice's physician shareholder/owners as compensation and fringe benefits. It is a single measurement that recognizes the net effect for any activity, in that a change in either revenue or operating expense will be reflected in revenue after operating cost. It represents the "bottom line" measure of practice performance.

■ HOW DO PRACTICES STAFF?

Medical practices exhibit high variability in their staffing strategies. An assessment of the staffing ratios reported by the medical groups that responded to the MGMA *Cost Survey: 2001 Report Based on 2000 Data* is provided in this chapter. The staffing levels reported by multispecialty groups with primary and specialty care, multispecialty groups with primary care only, family practice, cardiology, obstetrics and gynecology, and orthopedic surgery single specialty groups are reported in Graphs 3.1a, 3.2a, 3.3a, 3.4a, 3.5a, and 3.6a, respectively. To keep the data homogeneous, medical groups that were owned by hospitals were excluded from this analysis.

Examining the graphs suggests:

- There is a pattern in how medical groups staff;
- Different specialties staff at different levels;
- Staffing levels generally are distributed to resemble a "bell-shaped curve;"
- Some practices staff at much higher or much lower levels than others in the same specialty; and
- Staffing and profitability are related.

To better understand how to interpret the graphs, examine Figure 3.4a and note how the staffing level distribution varies for family practice single-specialty groups. This bar graph displays the distribution of different levels of staffing for the 50 family practice groups that responded to the MGMA *Cost Survey: 2001 Report Based on 2000 Data* and were not owned by a hospital or integrated delivery system. Staffing is measured as the total number of full-time equivalent (FTE) employees per FTE physician, categorized into 1.00 FTE employee ranges. The median for FTE employees per FTE physician for all family practice groups is 4.67, which occurs in the range with the longest bar on the graph. The bar graph shows that 42 percent of the responding practices had relatively similar staffing clustered at the midpoint. The bar graph also shows that there is substantial variance in staffing among the responding practices. Some practices have as few as 2.5 to 3.4 staff per doctor, while others are in the range of 8.5 to 9.4 FTE employees per FTE physician. These data indicate that there is substantial variation in staffing patterns among these family practice medical groups.

■ UNDERSTANDING CONSTRAINTS

To best measure the rightsize of staff for a medical group, it is necessary to understand the general functions the staff members perform. In this macro-level analysis of overall staffing levels, staff functions can be summarized as (1) functions that enable the physicians and other providers in patient treatment and (2) functions that perform the administrative tasks necessary to sustain the practice. While this description may appear simplistic, it lets one readily understand that the staff's core function is to optimize the productivity of the group's physicians and other providers, and its secondary responsibility is to sustain the day-to-day and long-term operation of the practice.

Physician (and other provider) time is the constraint that significantly limits the performance of a medical group relative to its goal of maximizing practice revenue. Medical groups that have successfully rightsized recognize the following advantages:

- Use of physician time is improved;
- Physicians are using their distinct competency and not performing tasks better relegated to support staff;
- Physicians are enabled to perform their patient care functions efficiently;
- Sources of delay or decreased output are removed; and
- Tasks best suited are delegated to trained, professional support staff, such as patient education, immunizations, wound dressing, etc.

The cost of physician time can be estimated by measuring the potential revenue that can be generated by the physician in an hour of patient care. This value will vary by specialty, but typically will range from $200 to $300 per hour. The rightsized practice recognizes that by increasing the number of staff, the constraint of physician time can be reduced and the increased expense in staff salary and benefits will be balanced by increased physician production. Since physician time has a very high value per hour, the increased production not only covers the higher salary and benefit cost associated with the additional staff; it also contributes additional revenue to the practice's bottom line.

Examining the constraints that prevent a medical practice from realizing its production potential is the best strategy to understand the rightsize for the practice's support staff. If physician time is the major constraint in production, a medical practice's level of performance can be improved by either extending the time the physician devotes to patient care, or making the time the physician spends in patient care more efficient. Many physicians have extended their workday, or they have extended their workweek to increase patient care time. This strategy has natural limitations and quickly reaches a level of diminishing return. The remaining option is for physicians to be more efficient in their use of time. Facility design is an important factor in increasing efficiency. Streamlined processes and procedures and the use of technology to increase production can also bring improvement. However, rightsizing staff to properly support the needs of the physician may be the easiest to implement, quickest to realize payback and least expensive solution to maximizing the time physicians spend in patient care.

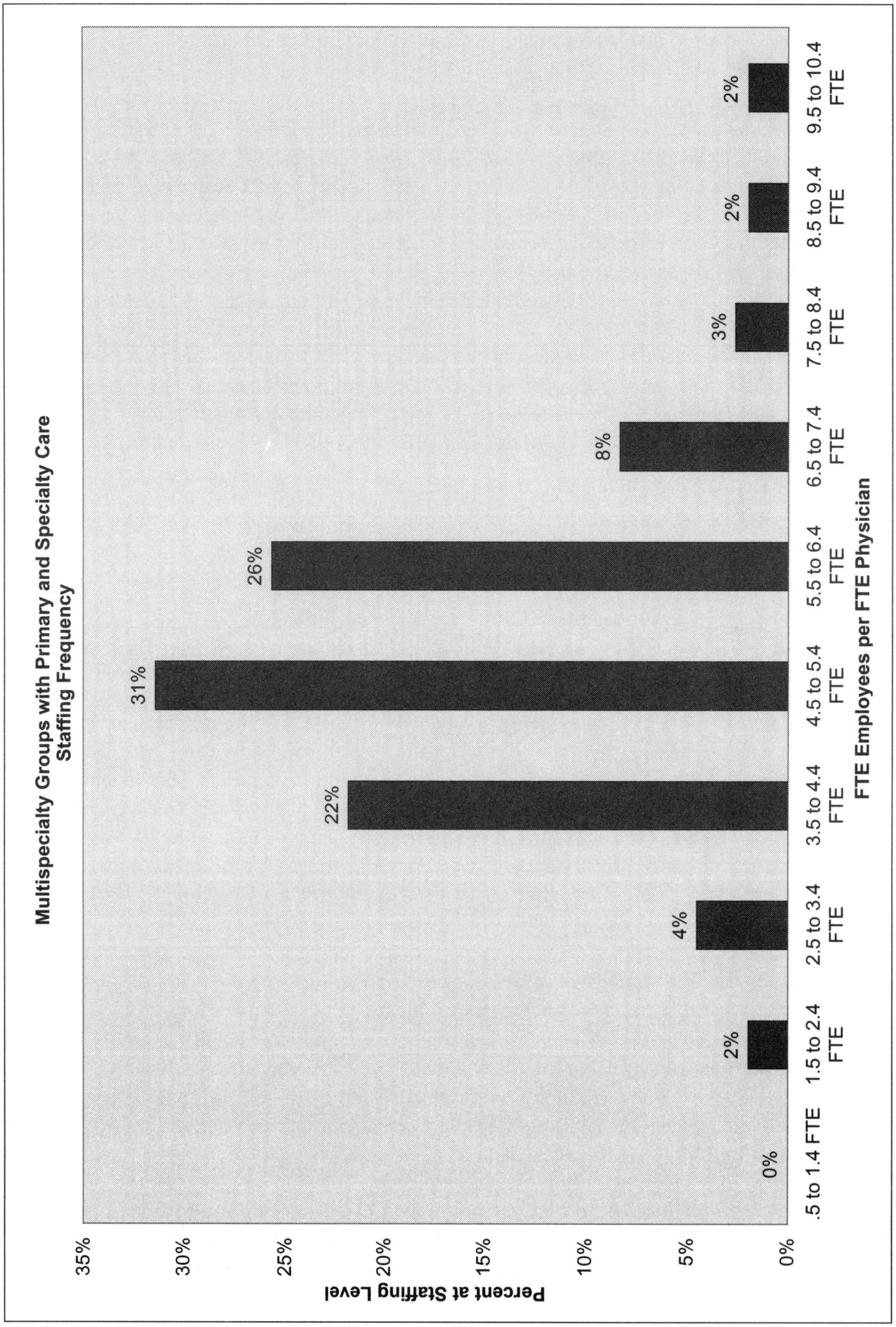

14 ■ CHAPTER 3

Multispecialty Groups with Primary and Specialty Care Staffing Frequency

FTE Employees per FTE Physician	Percent at Staffing Level
.5 to 1.4 FTE	0%
1.5 to 2.4 FTE	2%
2.5 to 3.4 FTE	4%
3.5 to 4.4 FTE	22%
4.5 to 5.4 FTE	31%
5.5 to 6.4 FTE	26%
6.5 to 7.4 FTE	8%
7.5 to 8.4 FTE	3%
8.5 to 9.4 FTE	2%
9.5 to 10.4 FTE	2%

GRAPH 3.1A ■

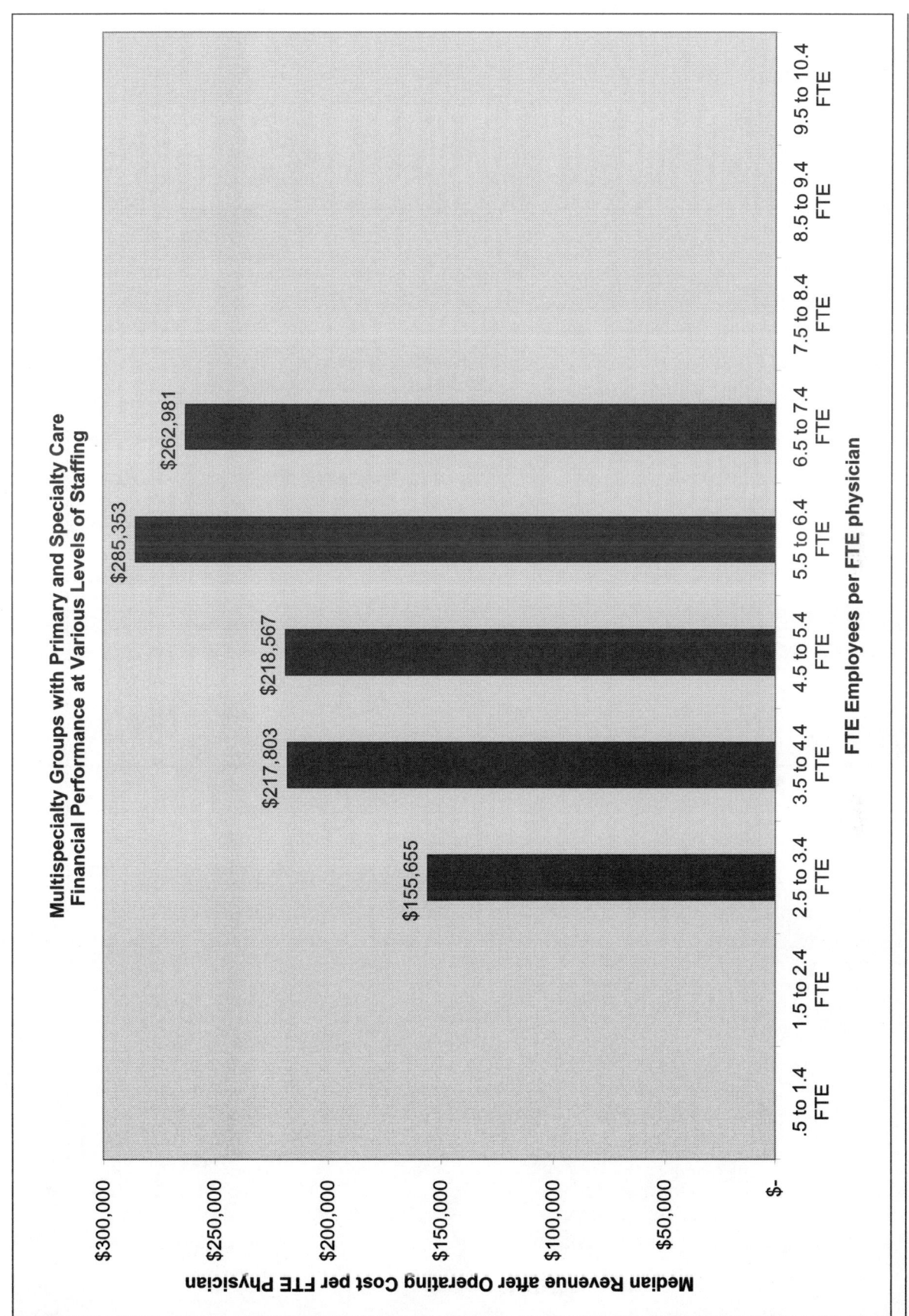

How Staffing Levels Affect Medical Practice Profitability 15

**Multispecialty Groups with Primary and Specialty Care
Financial Performance at Various Levels of Staffing**

FTE Employees per FTE physician	Median Revenue after Operating Cost per FTE Physician
.5 to 1.4 FTE	—
1.5 to 2.4 FTE	—
2.5 to 3.4 FTE	$155,655
3.5 to 4.4 FTE	$217,803
4.5 to 5.4 FTE	$218,567
5.5 to 6.4 FTE	$285,353
6.5 to 7.4 FTE	$262,981
7.5 to 8.4 FTE	—
8.5 to 9.4 FTE	—
9.5 to 10.4 FTE	—

GRAPH 3.1B

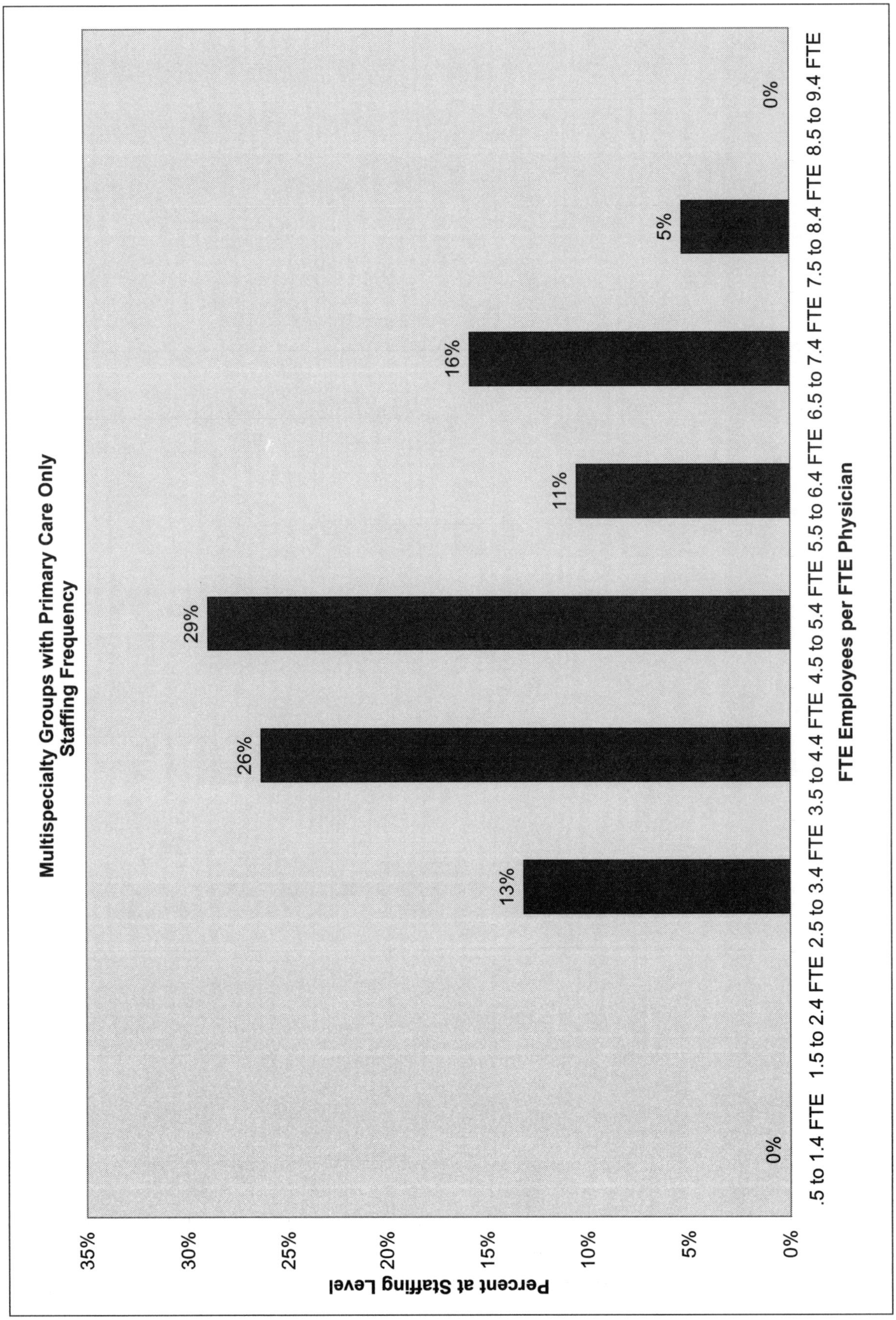

16 ◼ CHAPTER 3

**Multispecialty Groups with Primary Care Only
Staffing Frequency**

FTE Employees per FTE Physician	Percent at Staffing Level
.5 to 1.4 FTE	0%
1.5 to 2.4 FTE	13%
2.5 to 3.4 FTE	26%
3.5 to 4.4 FTE	29%
4.5 to 5.4 FTE	11%
5.5 to 6.4 FTE	16%
6.5 to 7.4 FTE	5%
7.5 to 8.4 FTE	0%
8.5 to 9.4 FTE	

GRAPH 3.2A ◼

How Staffing Levels Affect Medical Practice Profitability 17

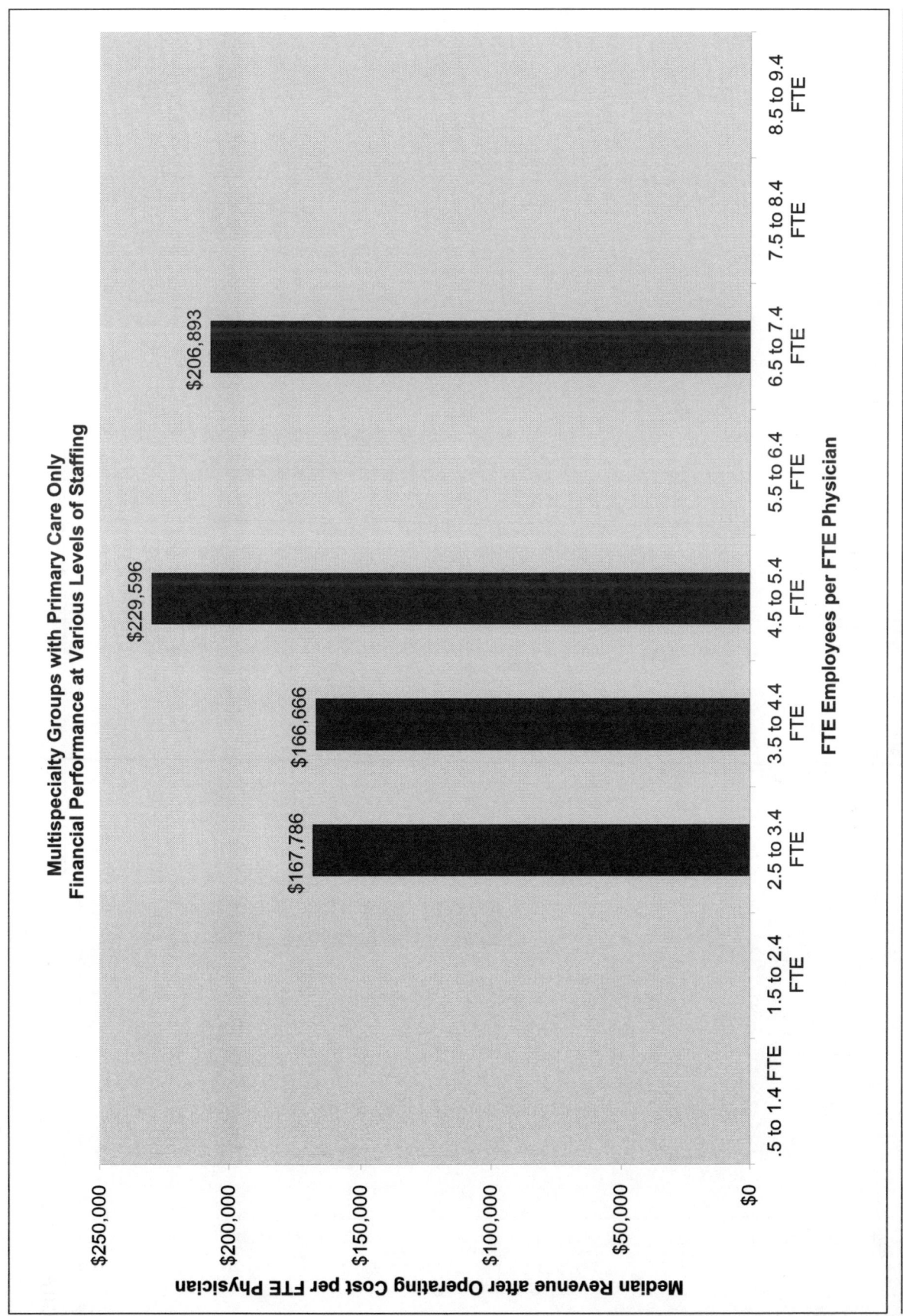

GRAPH 3.2B

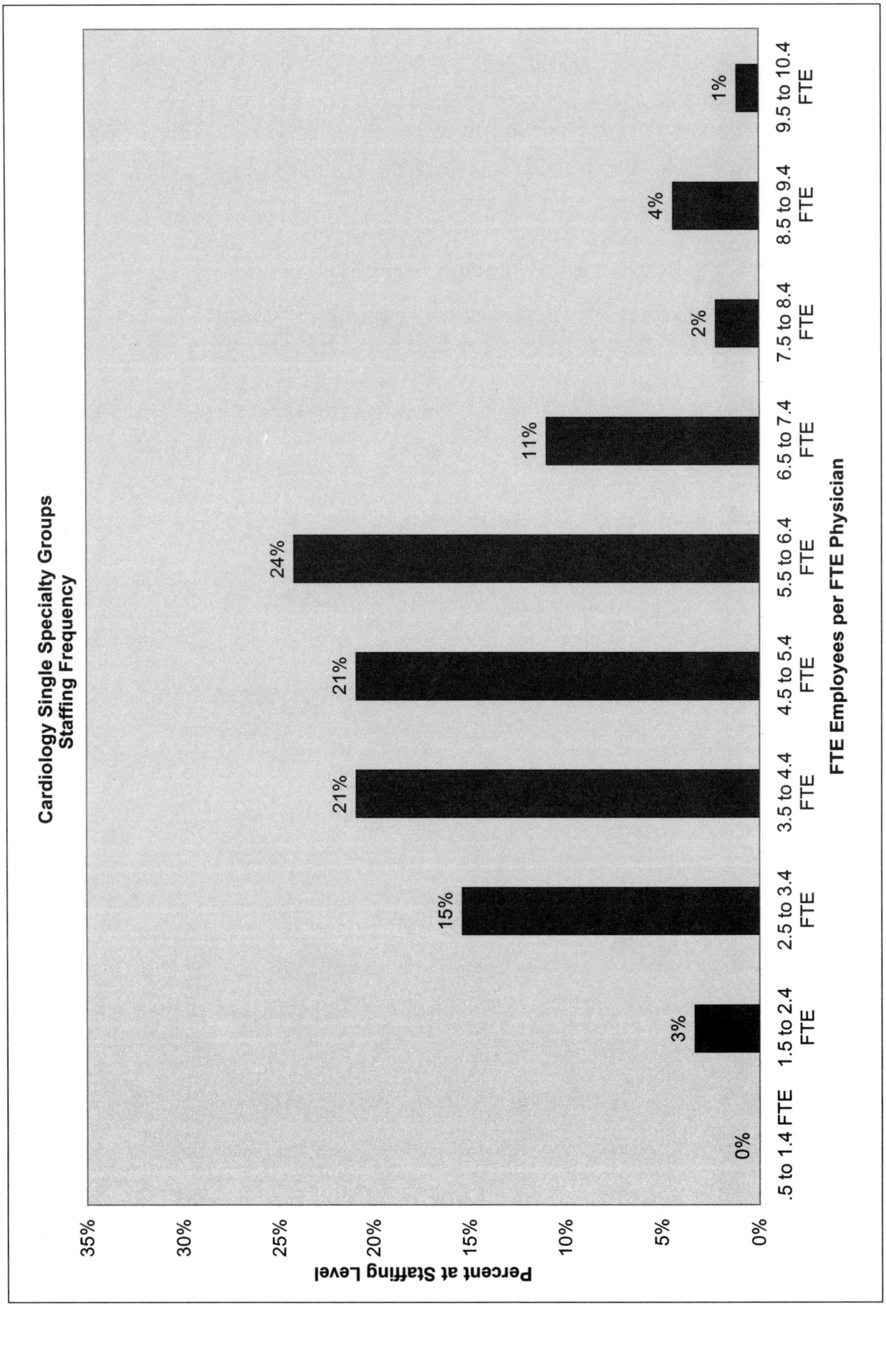

18 ■ CHAPTER 3

**Cardiology Single Specialty Groups
Staffing Frequency**

FTE Employees per FTE Physician	Percent at Staffing Level
.5 to 1.4 FTE	0%
1.5 to 2.4 FTE	3%
2.5 to 3.4 FTE	15%
3.5 to 4.4 FTE	21%
4.5 to 5.4 FTE	21%
5.5 to 6.4 FTE	24%
6.5 to 7.4 FTE	11%
7.5 to 8.4 FTE	2%
8.5 to 9.4 FTE	4%
9.5 to 10.4 FTE	1%

GRAPH 3.3A ■

How Staffing Levels Affect Medical Practice Profitability ■ 19

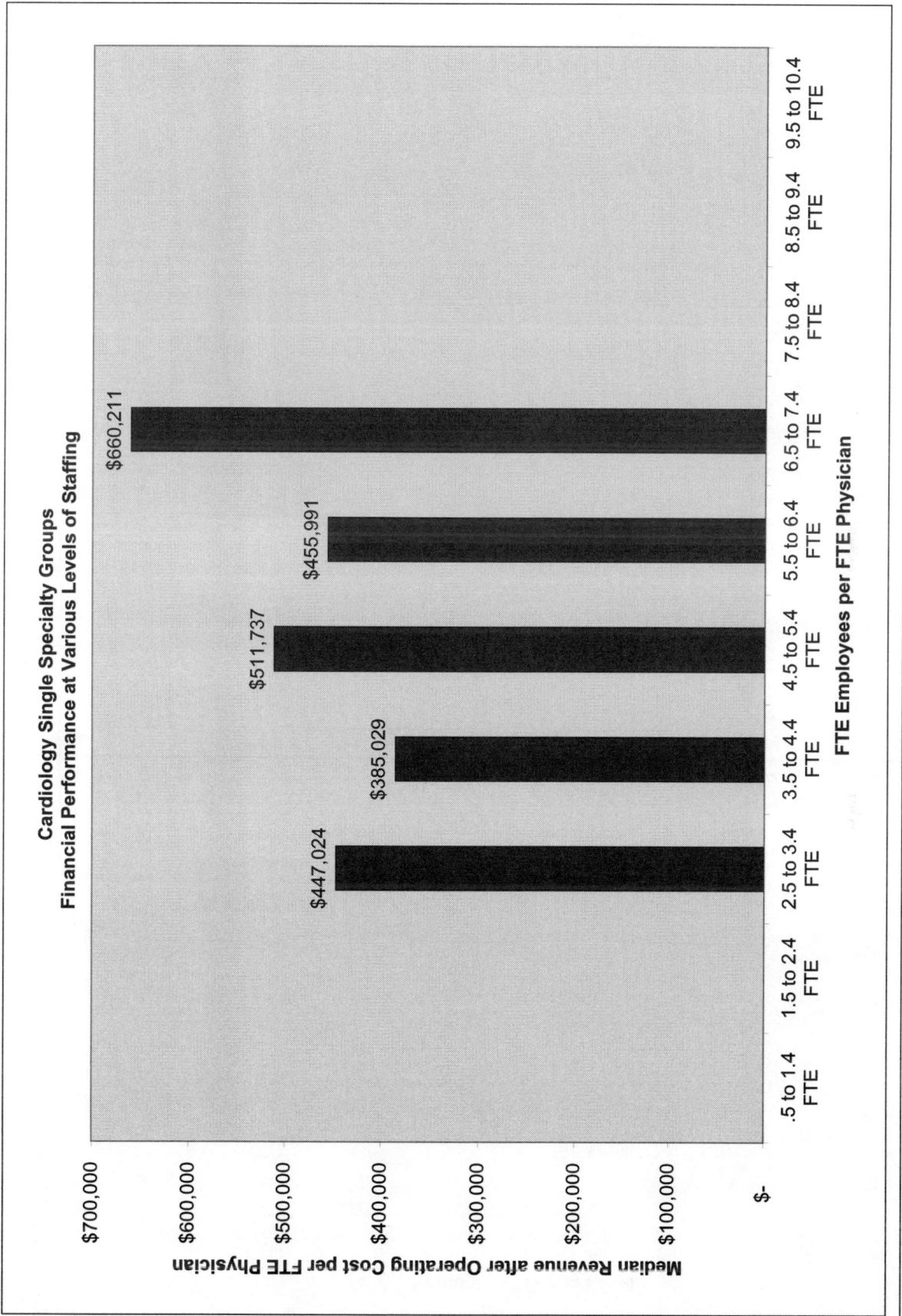

GRAPH 3.3B

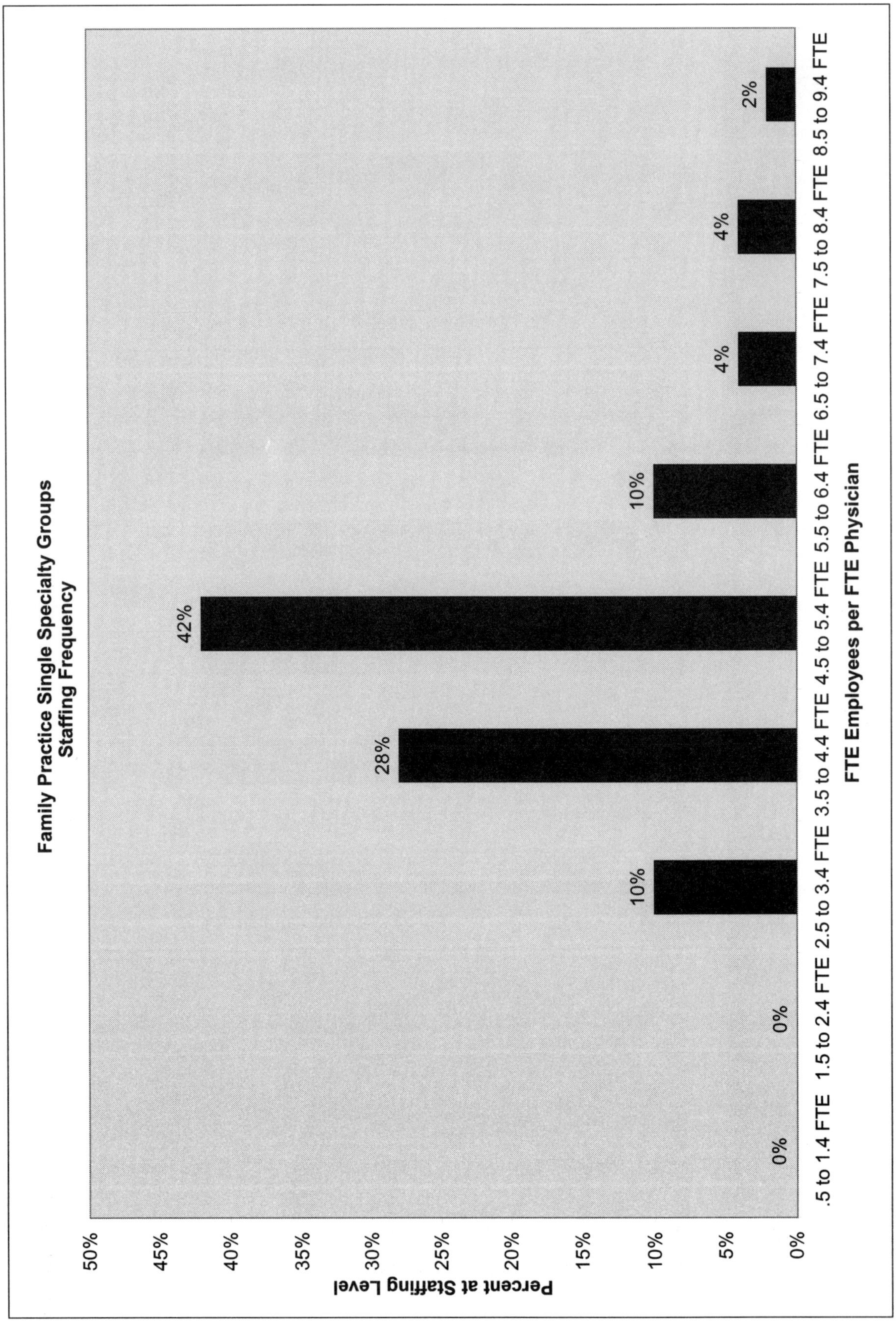

20 ■ CHAPTER 3

**Family Practice Single Specialty Groups
Staffing Frequency**

FTE Employees per FTE Physician	Percent at Staffing Level
.5 to 1.4 FTE	0%
1.5 to 2.4 FTE	0%
2.5 to 3.4 FTE	10%
3.5 to 4.4 FTE	28%
4.5 to 5.4 FTE	42%
5.5 to 6.4 FTE	10%
6.5 to 7.4 FTE	4%
7.5 to 8.4 FTE	4%
8.5 to 9.4 FTE	2%

GRAPH 3.4A ■

How Staffing Levels Affect Medical Practice Profitability ■ 21

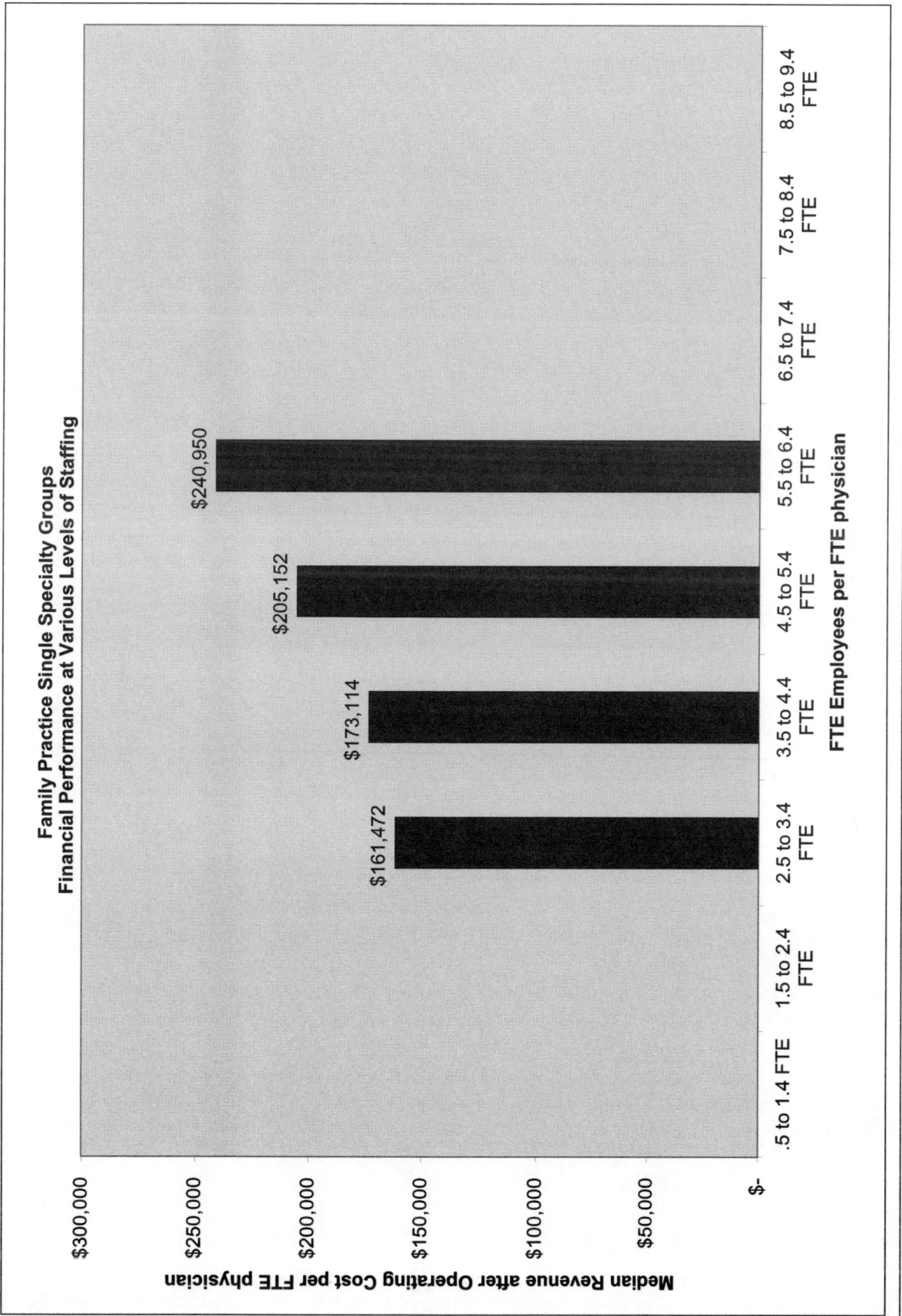

GRAPH 3.4B ■

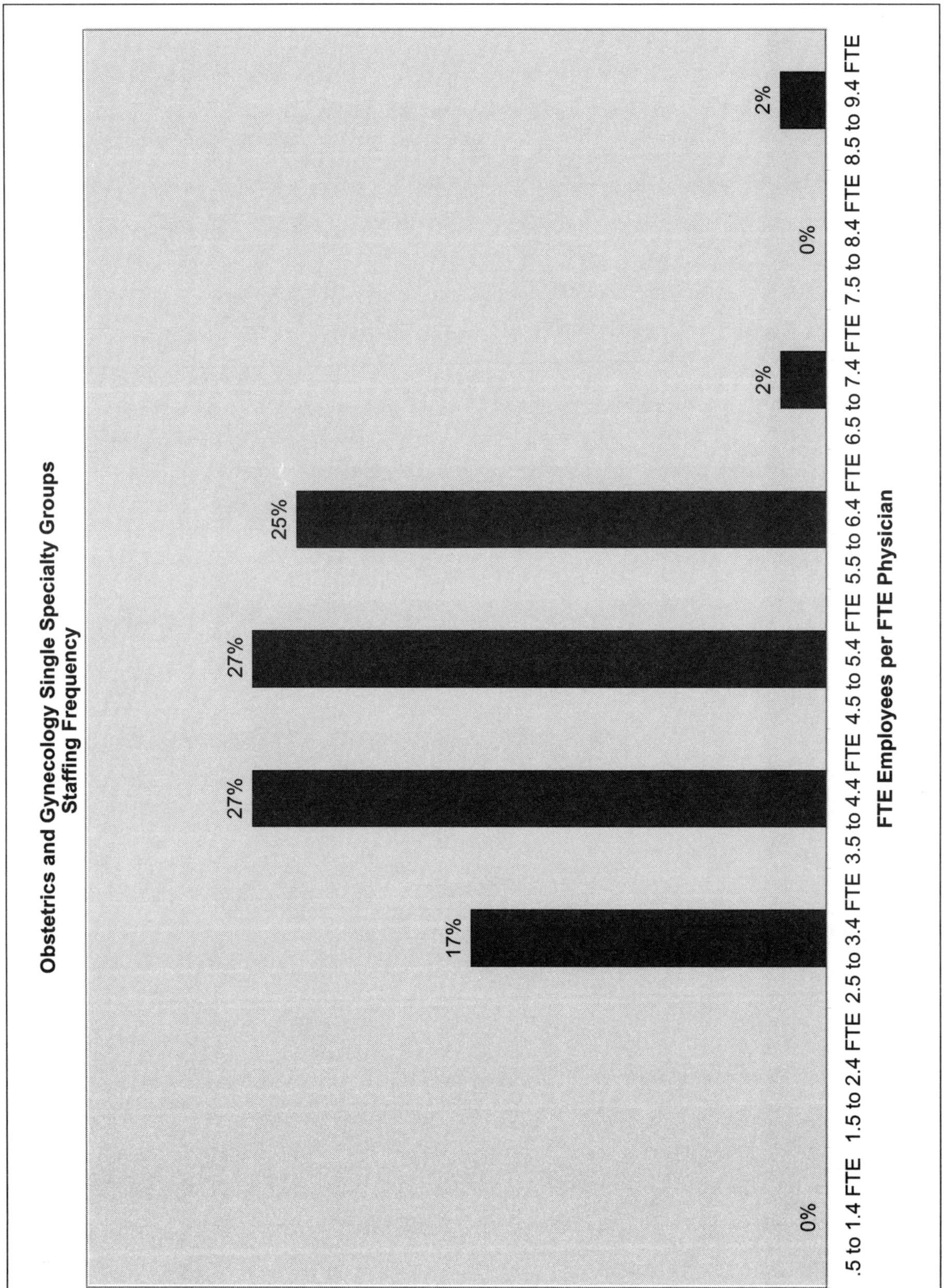

22 ■ CHAPTER 3

**Obstetrics and Gynecology Single Specialty Groups
Staffing Frequency**

FTE Employees per FTE Physician	Percent with Staffing Level
.5 to 1.4 FTE	0%
1.5 to 2.4 FTE	17%
2.5 to 3.4 FTE	27%
3.5 to 4.4 FTE	27%
4.5 to 5.4 FTE	25%
5.5 to 6.4 FTE	2%
6.5 to 7.4 FTE	0%
7.5 to 8.4 FTE	0%
8.5 to 9.4 FTE	2%

GRAPH 3.5A ■

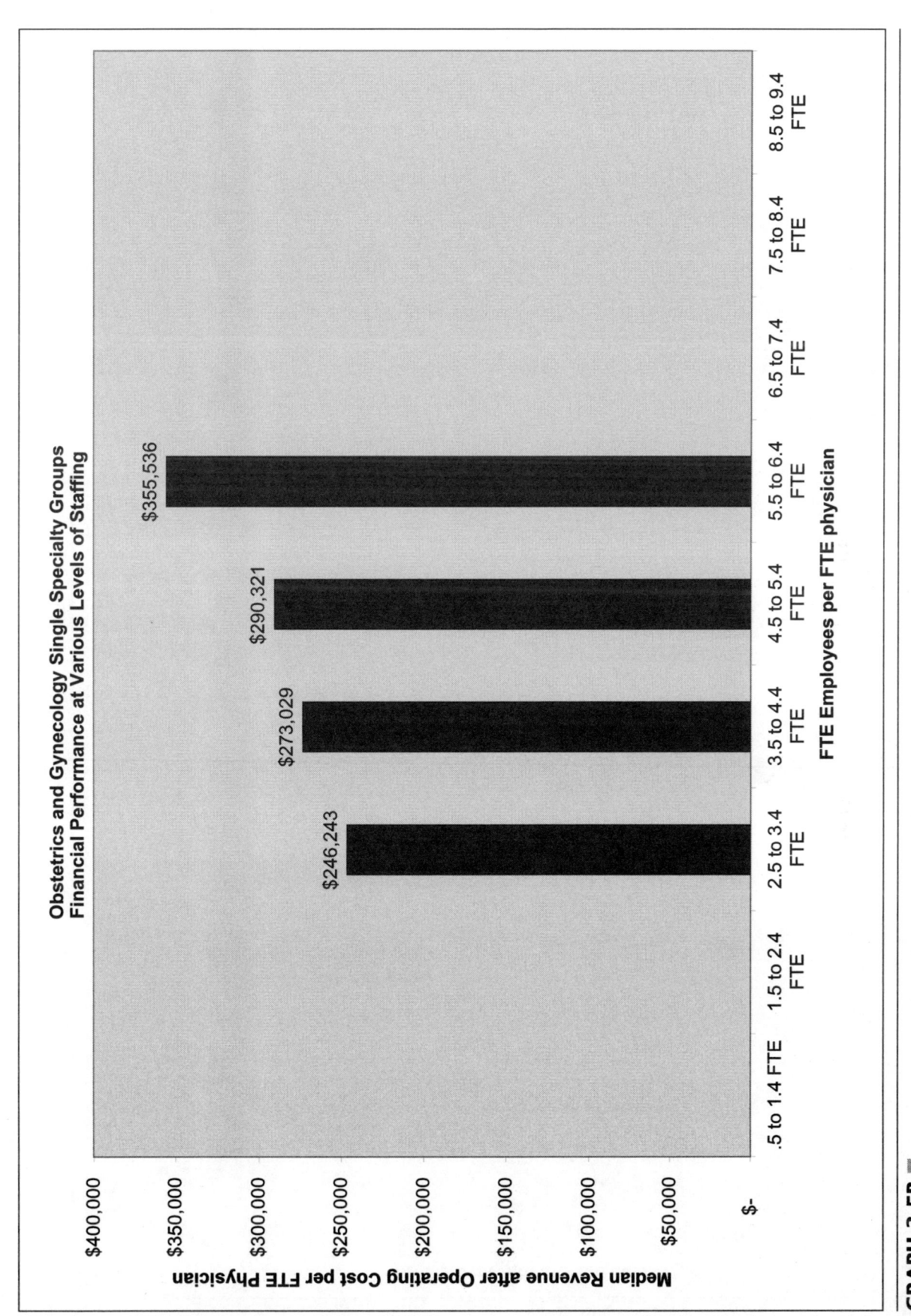

How Staffing Levels Affect Medical Practice Profitability ■ 23

Obstetrics and Gynecology Single Specialty Groups
Financial Performance at Various Levels of Staffing

FTE Employees per FTE physician	Median Revenue after Operating Cost per FTE Physician
.5 to 1.4 FTE	—
1.5 to 2.4 FTE	—
2.5 to 3.4 FTE	$246,243
3.5 to 4.4 FTE	$273,029
4.5 to 5.4 FTE	$290,321
5.5 to 6.4 FTE	$355,536
6.5 to 7.4 FTE	—
7.5 to 8.4 FTE	—
8.5 to 9.4 FTE	—

GRAPH 3.5B ■

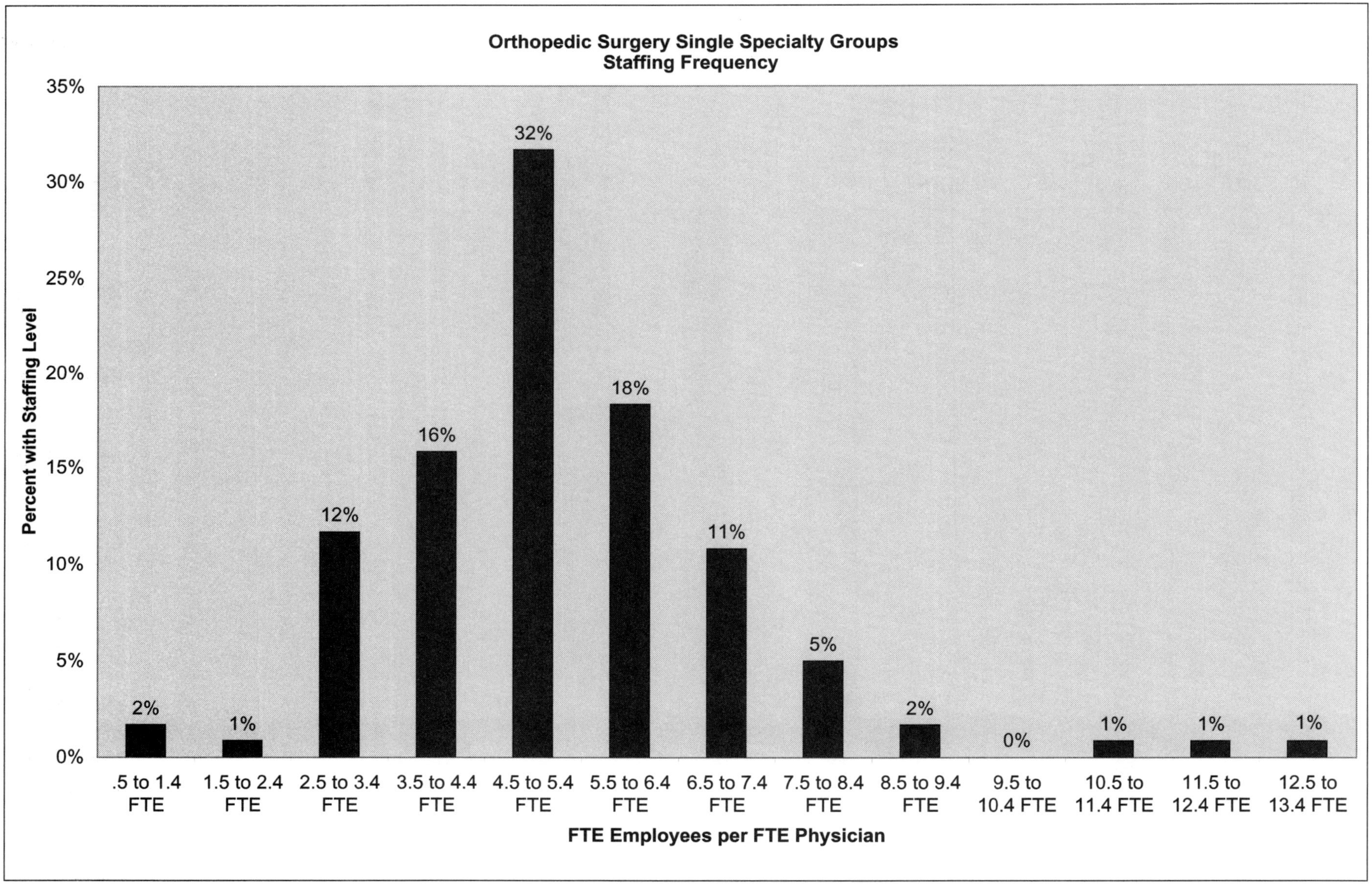

Orthopedic Surgery Single Specialty Groups
Staffing Frequency

FTE Employees per FTE Physician	Percent with Staffing Level
.5 to 1.4 FTE	2%
1.5 to 2.4 FTE	1%
2.5 to 3.4 FTE	12%
3.5 to 4.4 FTE	16%
4.5 to 5.4 FTE	32%
5.5 to 6.4 FTE	18%
6.5 to 7.4 FTE	11%
7.5 to 8.4 FTE	5%
8.5 to 9.4 FTE	2%
9.5 to 10.4 FTE	0%
10.5 to 11.4 FTE	1%
11.5 to 12.4 FTE	1%
12.5 to 13.4 FTE	1%

GRAPH 3.6A

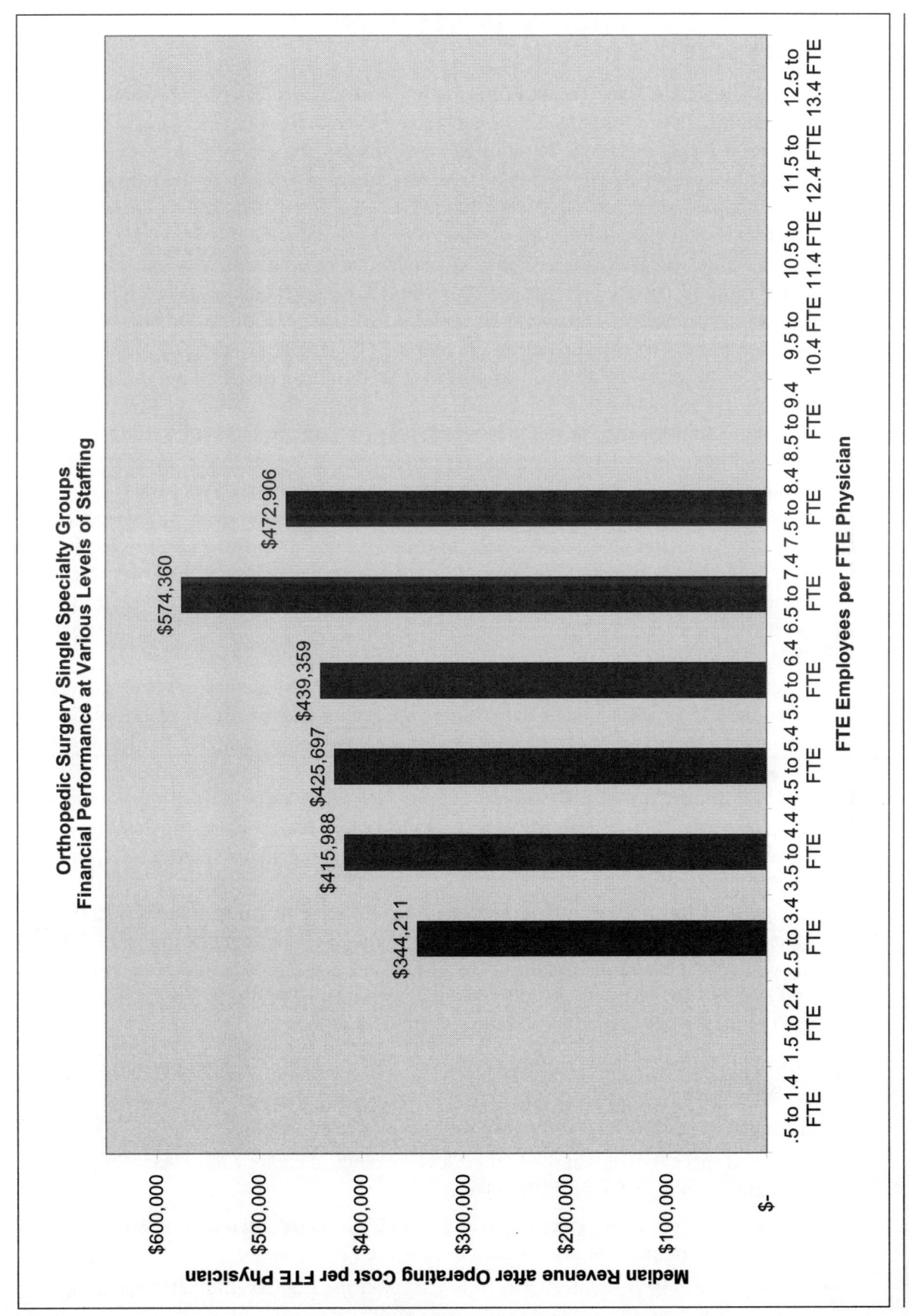

How Staffing Levels Affect Medical Practice Profitability ■ 25

Orthopedic Surgery Single Specialty Groups
Financial Performance at Various Levels of Staffing

FTE Employees per FTE Physician	Median Revenue after Operating Cost per FTE Physician
.5 to 1.4 FTE	$344,211
1.5 to 2.4 FTE	$415,988
2.5 to 3.4 FTE	$425,697
3.5 to 4.4 FTE	$439,359
4.5 to 5.4 FTE	
5.5 to 6.4 FTE	$574,360
6.5 to 7.4 FTE	$472,906
7.5 to 8.4 FTE	
8.5 to 9.4 FTE	
9.5 to 10.4 FTE	
10.5 to 11.4 FTE	
11.5 to 12.4 FTE	
12.5 to 13.4 FTE	

GRAPH 3.6B ■

INCREASED PROFITABILITY IS ASSOCIATED WITH RIGHTSIZED STAFFING

The same database that provides information on how medical practices staff also provides insight into how different staffing levels affect the practice's bottom line financial success. Graphs 3.1b, 3.2b, 3.3b, 3.4b, 3.5b and 3.6b display the amount of medical revenue after operating cost per FTE physician at the same ranges of staffing as the bar graphs that depict the frequency of staffing at each level. These graphs display the financial benefits that result from the various levels of staffing. (For statistical reliability and confidentiality, data were suppressed when there were fewer than five respondents in a category, so not every staffing level depicted on the first bar graph also has financial data displayed.) For each practice, the medical revenue after operating cost per FTE physician was calculated. The practices were then categorized by the ratio of FTE Employees per FTE physician, and the median, or midpoint value, was computed for each staffing category and is displayed on the graphs.

The graphs indicate that, at the lowest and often the highest levels of staffing, practices generally reported lower levels of financial performance. At the lower levels of staffing, physician production is, most likely, constrained, which results in lower production and lower total medical revenue than that reported by other practices. Even though personnel costs and general operating costs are lower for these practices (not shown on the graphs, but observed in the raw data), total revenue and revenue after operating cost are lower since production is constrained. A different situation occurs at the highest levels of staffing. The increased cost of staff exceeds the increase in revenue realized from higher production; therefore, the amount of medical revenue after operating cost decreases.

In general, these graphs illustrate that the highest levels of medical revenue after operating cost per FTE physician occur when there are higher levels of staffing, but not at the absolute highest ratio. For family practice single specialty groups, Graph 3.4b illustrates that the lowest level of medical revenue after operating cost per FTE physician occurs at the lowest level of staffing, 2.5 to 3.4 FTE employees per FTE physician, and medical revenue after operating cost per FTE physician increases at each staffing level. The staffing category with the highest medical revenue after operating cost per FTE physician is 5.5 to 6.4 FTE employees per FTE physician.

This peak on the graph can be interpreted to coincide with the rightsize for staffing in the specialty. This observation is consistent with the concept that the rightsize level of staffing will offset constraints that limit the physician's capacity to see patients in the practice and is supported by the increased revenue that results from higher productivity.

The financial performance graphs support these observations:

- There is a pattern in how staffing levels affect medical revenue after operating cost per FTE physician;
- Different specialties have different levels of financial performance;
- Different specialties obtain the highest level of medical revenue after operating cost per FTE physician at different staffing levels;
- Medical revenue after operating cost per FTE physician increases as staffing levels increase to a point where rightsizing occurs, then it decreases; and
- Some practices have much higher or much lower medical revenue after operating cost per FTE physician than others in the same specialty.

APPLYING GENERAL PERFORMANCE INFORMATION TO A SPECIFIC PRACTICE

The findings of this study must be interpreted in the unique context of each practice. The graphs display the general changes in medical revenue after operating cost per FTE physician that occur in a number of practices and demonstrate that this value can change at different staffing levels.

It should be noted that the staffing level is only one factor that could affect practice profitability. As stated earlier, other factors such as physician practice style, group culture, competitive market factors, facility layout, scheduling methods and technology can also affect profitability. Importantly, patient demand and patient health status will impact staffing requirements and physician time. In addition, profitability is directly related to payer mix and reimbursement levels, measures for which the practice has only limited control.

The systematic approach to rightsizing the medical practice that is described in this text is designed to assist medical practice leaders and administrators in identifying opportunities to rightsize staffing that will have a positive contribution to the practice's profitability, as well as to practice productivity and efficiency. Employees are a medical practice's most valuable resource and the basis for a practice's ultimate success. Rightsizing the staffing level in a medical group is critical to achieving its financial goals and to providing high quality, patient-focused, health care services.

A practice's unique situation will determine its rightsize and the data referenced in this chapter provide evidence of staffing impact on profitability. Through a systematic approach to staff rightsizing, a medical practice can determine its appropriate staffing levels.

CHAPTER 4

Staffing Is a Measure of Work

■ LINKING STAFF TO PHYSICIAN WORK LEVELS

The key to efficient staffing models and staffing deployment is to recognize that staffing is a measure of work. That is, the volume of staff and the skill mix of staff vary based upon physician and practice work levels. Historically, many practices have attempted to provide the same number of nurses or the same number of medical assistants to each physician working in the practice. Physicians exhibit different levels of productivity and perform different scopes of service which, in turn, may require different levels of staff support. The historical staffing models have been supplanted by newer approaches that assign staff based upon physician work levels, with many medical practices adopting staffing models involving shared or centralized staff support functions.

The impact of the physician's specialty, productivity, scope of service delivery and other similar factors on the rightsizing process will now be explored.

■ IMPACT OF MEDICAL OR SURGICAL SPECIALTY ON STAFFING

Different levels of staffing in a medical practice are needed, depending upon the physician's specialty. For example, primary care practices will have more support staff than surgical practices since most of the work conducted by the primary care physician is in the office setting rather than in the hospital. As an example, family practice single specialty groups report a median of 4.67 FTE support staff per FTE physician, while general surgery single specialty groups report 2.89 FTE support staff per FTE physician (MGMA *Cost Survey: 2001 Report Based on 2000 Data*). Similarly, multispecialty practices that only provide primary care services will reflect higher staffing levels than multispecialty practices that provide both primary and specialty care due to the preponderance of activity conducted in the medical practice's outpatient setting.

Beyond simply the volume of staff deployed in the outpatient setting, staffing cost per physician and staffing cost as a percent of total medical revenue will obviously be different among different medical and surgical specialties due to variation in medical revenue generating capability. Family practice single specialty medical groups, for example, report a median cost of $139,054 support staff cost per FTE physician and a median support staff cost as a percent of total medical revenue of 31.57 percent. General surgery single specialty practices, on the other hand, report $113,837 median support staff cost per FTE physician, with a median staff cost as a percent of total medical revenue of 20.64 percent (MGMA *Cost Survey: 2001 Report Based on 2000 Data*).

■ IMPACT OF PHYSICIAN PRODUCTIVITY AND PRACTICE SCOPE ON STAFFING

The scope of services provided by the physician and the productivity of the physician will also impact staffing since staffing is a measure of work. The MGMA Cost Survey data suggest a relationship between the number of clinical and ancillary staff per FTE physician and both total procedures performed and total medical revenue generated per FTE physician. The following scatterplots demonstrate this relationship.

In Graph 4.1, the x-axis reflects total clinical and ancillary staff per FTE physician, with the y-axis reporting total procedures per FTE physician for multispecialty practices with primary care only. The R^2 of .33 indicates that 33 percent of the change in total procedures per FTE physician is attributed to the number of clinical and ancillary staff per FTE physician employed in the practice. Similarly, as demonstrated in Graph 4.2, clinical and ancillary staff per FTE physician explains 44 percent of the change in total medical revenue per FTE physician. This association between total clinical and ancillary support staff and total procedures and total medical revenue is also found among family practice single specialty groups. In these groups, as demonstrated in Graph 4.3 and in Graph 4.4, 25 percent and 33

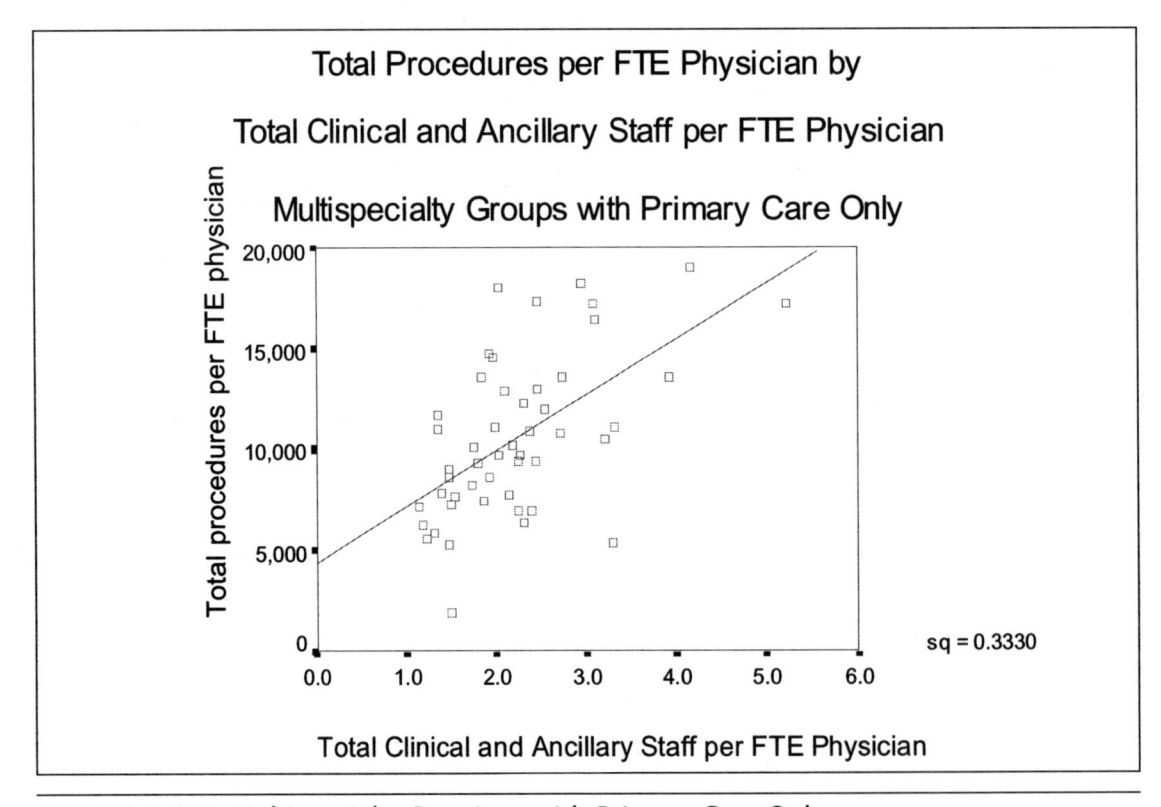

GRAPH 4.1 ■ Multispecialty Practices with Primary Care Only

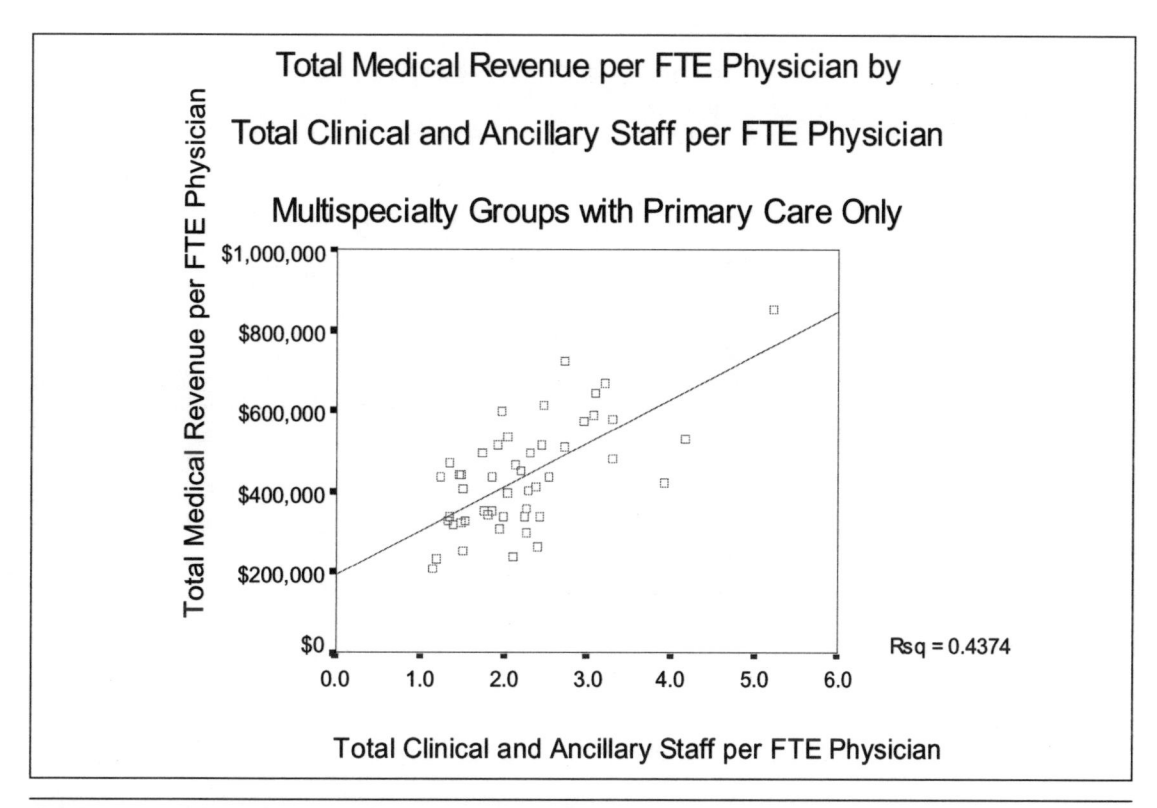

Staffing Is a Measure of Work ■ 31

Total Medical Revenue per FTE Physician by Total Clinical and Ancillary Staff per FTE Physician

Multispecialty Groups with Primary Care Only

Rsq = 0.4374

GRAPH 4.2 ■ Multispecialty Practices with Primary Care Only

Total Procedures per FTE Physician by Total Clinical and Ancillary Staff per FTE Physician

Family Practice

sq = 0.2490

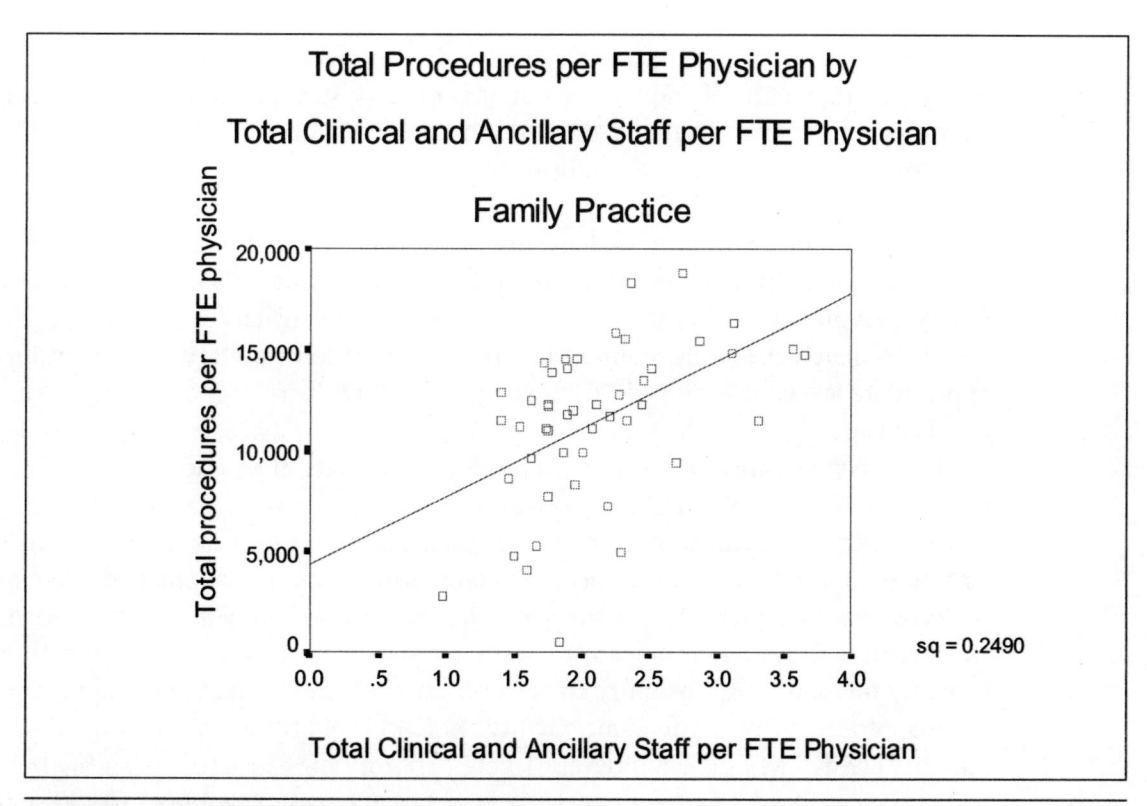

GRAPH 4.3 ■ Family Practice Single Specialty

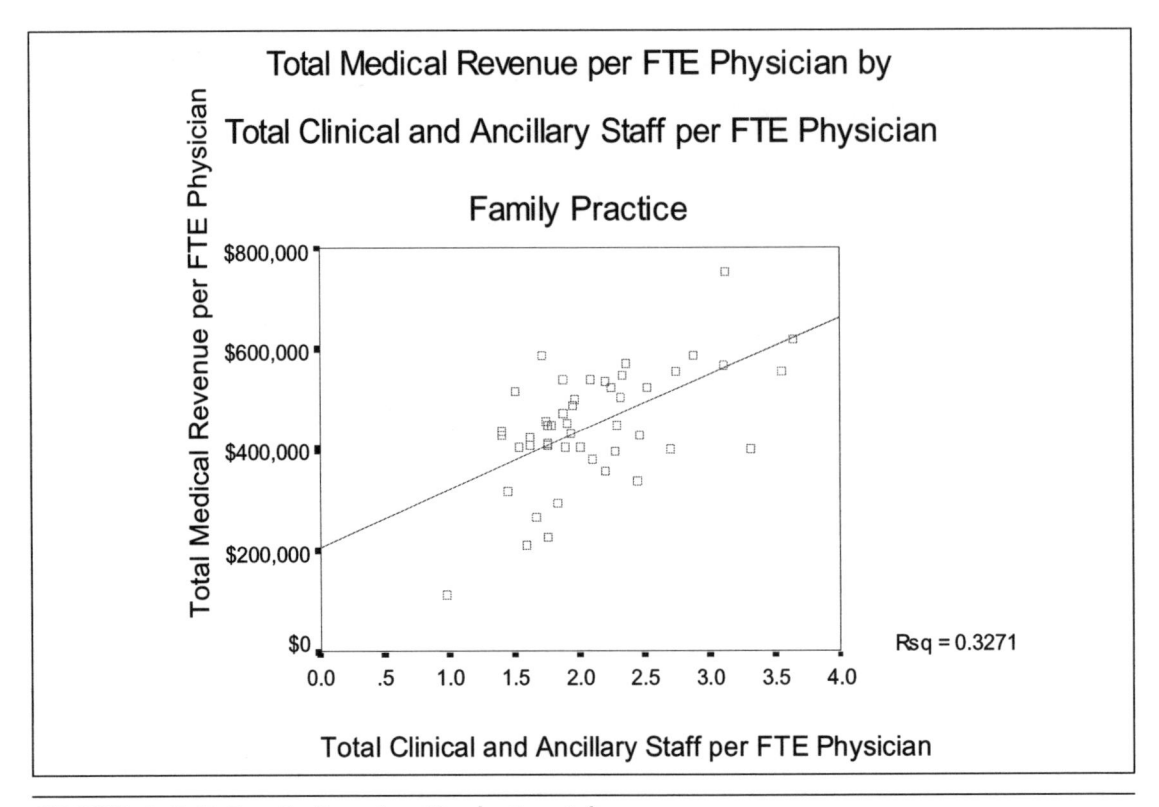

Total Medical Revenue per FTE Physician by Total Clinical and Ancillary Staff per FTE Physician

Family Practice

Rsq = 0.3271

GRAPH 4.4 ■ Family Practice Single Specialty

percent of the change in total procedures and total medical revenue, respectively, is attributed to the total clinical and ancillary staff per FTE physician employed in the practice. The data support the concept that staffing is a measure of work.

A match of the employee's skills to the actual work that needs to be performed in the medical practice is also required for appropriate rightsizing of the practice. Utilizing a registered nurse simply to room patients and function as a medical assistant is not a good use of resources for the practice. Similarly, if a medical assistant is asked to perform nursing duties, that model would present a business risk and potentially impact quality of care. The goal is to match the skills required for the particular job function or task and to delegate appropriate levels of responsibility to support staff within the scope of their classification and licensure.

If physicians perform at very high productivity levels, then additional staff may be warranted based upon these high levels (however, the skill mix of staff would also need to be assessed). An identical staffing model for each physician that does not take into account variation in productivity will be inefficient and costly for a practice. The number of patients seen by a physician in the outpatient setting will depend upon hours of practice, the scheduling model employed, the efficiency of the provider, the degree to which the provider delegates responsibility to the clinical staff, the market and the practice culture, among others. Within the same facility, however, a physician electing to see only 18 patients per day will need a different level of staffing infrastructure than his/her colleague who regularly sees 32 patients per day. These variable patient volumes would suggest a different staffing infrastructure to support not only the in-office patient flow process, but also the telephone management, nurse triage, prescription refill processes and test results reporting processes that are associated with the physician's patient panel size.

Based upon MGMA data, the numbers in Figure 4.1 are provided as a guide to evaluate physician productivity in the medical practice (data reflect annual volumes). Assuming 48 weeks per year at 4.5 days per week, a daily production volume can be computed; however, an analysis of financial performance would also be needed to determine if these productivity levels support an appropriate financial position for the group.

Using physician production data, a practice can compute its staff cost per Work Relative Value Units (WRVU) and staff hours per WRVU, providing a comparative analysis among its practice sites relative to skill mix requirements to support practice workload variation.

Many practices that analyze staffing based on a physician's panel size further adjust the panel size by patient age, gender and other risk factors to determine the workload associated with a physician's panel. As a proxy for patient panel size, unique visit counts for the past 12 to 24 month period may be used to identify the variable workloads among physicians and to investigate the need for variable staffing levels and skill mix to support clinical activity.

The presence or absence of two other programs, in particular, will also impact physician productivity and staffing levels: 1) hospitalists and 2) immediate or urgent care capability.

1. Hospitalists

Availability of hospitalists typically permits a primary care physician to expand office hours by 8 to 9 hours per week, thereby permitting enhanced patient access and higher patient visit volumes. Staffing levels need to be consistent with these expanded hours and expanded physician productivity.

2. Immediate Care or Urgent Care Facility

The availability of an immediate care or urgent care facility impacts patient volume for primary care physicians (and may lessen continuity of care for patients). If patients

FIGURE 4.1 ■ Physician Productivity Measures

Specialty	Ambulatory Encounters	Hospital Encounters	Surgery/Anesthesia Cases	Work Relative Value Units
Family Practice (w/o OB)	4,396–5,446	347–631	270–545	3,834–4,631
General Internal Medicine	3,541–4,398	665–1139	197–607	3,790–4,565
Pediatrics	4,618–5,608	314–485	126–245	3,961–4,862
OB/GYN	3,029–3,818	127–259	435–684	6,123–7,576
Cardiology (Noninvasive)	2,044–3,613	1,365–2,032	200–304	6,221–8,112
Gastroenterology	1,550–2,260	798–1280	1,384–1,761	6,964–8,140
General Surgery	1,638–2,153	328–546	702–955	6,284–7,691
Orthopedic Surgery	3,425–4,229	111–171	493–869	7,014–8,756
Urology	2,995–3,702	232–362	936–1151	6,154–7,741

Source: MGMA *Physician Compensation & Production Survey: 2001 Report Based on 2000 Data.* Median to 75th percentile reported. Note: the above data represent only a small subset of this database which reports up to 105 specialties.

can self-select to the immediate care facility, physicians working in the scheduled office setting may see more difficult cases than their physician counterparts who practice in settings that do not have immediate care facilities. Additionally, with urgent care capability, physicians, nurses or scheduling staff may divert patients to the urgent care facility during the day or toward the end of office hours. This can have an impact on the volume of patients that are worked in to the schedule during the day to be seen by their physicians, thus impacting clinical productivity.

A walk-in facility co-located with a scheduled physician practice will also impact staffing workload and practice efficiency, since there is no opportunity to pre-plan for a walk-in patient visit. In a walk-in setting, the following types of activities need to be performed at the time of patient arrival, essentially in "real time," rather than be conducted as part of the planned pre-visit functions:

- Nurse triage;
- Updates to insurance and demographic information;
- Pre-authorization for services;
- Medical records retrieval;
- Medical records, charge ticket and other form preparation; and
- Activities associated with "anticipating the visit," for example, supplies, laboratory orders, etc.

It is important to understand the concept of "staffing is a measure of work." Rightsizing staff involves ensuring that staff performs at optimal levels with an appropriate delegation of breadth and scope of responsibility. Recognizing that staff is a measure of work, the practice must identify the skills needed by its staff based on the work to be performed and then (1) "match" staff to the required work functions and (2) ensure expected levels of productivity and performance are met.

The Impact of Internal Practice-Specific Factors on Rightsizing

CHAPTER 5

Data are used in the staff rightsizing methodology. It is important to recognize, however, that staffing levels are also determined by a host of internal, medical practice-specific factors that are qualitative in nature. Four key areas at the micro-system level of the medical practice that impact staff rightsizing will be discussed in this chapter:

1. **The practice model** that has been adopted;
2. **The patient scheduling methods** that are employed;
3. Limitations presented by the practice's physical space and **facility**; and
4. The practice's ability to **leverage technology**.

When consulting benchmark sources and interpreting the quantitative data, the impact of these practice-specific factors must be taken into account.

FIGURE 5.1 ■ Impact of Internal Medical Group Specific Factors on Rightsizing

1. Practice model
2. Patient scheduling methods
3. Practice facility
4. Technology

PRACTICE MODEL

As we will detail in the steps involved in rightsizing staff discussed in Chapter 6, an analysis of the practice model should be undertaken to determine if it is aligned with the goals and objectives of the medical practice. For purposes of this discussion, the term "practice model" will refer to the method by which the physicians have elected (or have been directed) to practice medicine. This encompasses a number of areas including:

- Whether the medical practice is organized as a true group practice (or simply individual practices that have been co-located);
- The number of practice sites in which physicians work;

- The skill mix of staff that has been requested or provided to the physician;
- The types of duties that have been delegated to the staff; and
- The extent to which specific tasks are shared or distributed.

One of the key advantages of a large multispecialty practice is the potential for economies of scale and scope. While no definitive medical practice size has been identified to maximize economies of scale, grouping or co-locating providers in 6 to 8 member clusters or suites tends to yield economies of scale that are not experienced by medical groups with smaller or larger-sized physician co-locations. Academic researchers investigating economies of scale in physician practices have estimated lowest cost practice size at 5.2 physicians;[8] however, they reported greatest office visit productivity in group practices of 3 or 4 physicians. In an earlier study researchers identified seven members as the most efficient scale of practice.[9] Thus, the size of the medical practice and the grouping of physicians in the practice's facility will impact the efficiency of the practice model.

Beyond size of practice considerations, the number of practice sites is also an important component of the practice model. If a medical group operates with more practice sites than its benchmark counterparts, its overall staffing levels and staffing on a per physician or per provider basis will likely be higher than benchmark norms.

The practice model that has been adopted will have a direct impact on staffing strategies employed in the medical practice. For example, for practices that have designated a one-to-one assignment of a nurse to a physician (with the nurse performing telephone nurse triage, managing the prescription refill process, managing test results reporting and other functions) the practice has limited alternatives when the nurse must be absent from work. Typically these practices secure registry staff or "float pool" staff to provide nursing coverage for the physician. A change to the practice model involving shared nurse triage or establishment of a nurse advice unit and the creation of systematic processes to manage prescription refills or test results reporting, for example, may permit a wider range of options for clinical support and may also serve to enhance patient service.

To illustrate the differences in staffing based on practice model, five different practice models are outlined in Table 5.1. As the variability of these models demonstrates, very different levels of front office (reception staff, telephone operators and patient scheduling staff) and clinical support staff (RN, LPN, and medical assistants) are required, depending upon the model that is embraced by the practice.

PRIMARY CARE A

In Primary Care A, each physician has been assigned his/her own registered nurse and medical assistant, consisting of a stand-alone, individual practice clinical support staff model. Non-clinical support staff is shared—that is, there are central patient check-in and patient check-out stations and central medical records. In this model, the registered nurse

---

[8]Pope GC and Burge RT. Economies of scale in physician practice. Medical Care Research and Review. December 1996; 53(4): 417-440.

[9]Kimbell L, Lorent J. Physician productivity and returns to scale. Health Services Research. Winter, 1977; 12(4): 367-380.

TABLE 5.1 ■ Examples of Practice Models

Primary Care A	Primary Care B	Primary Care C	Primary Care D	Primary Care E
RN & MA each	RN or LPN each	LPN or MA sharing of clinical support	RN each MA float	MA shared Central nurse triage
Central telephone scheduler/messages	Dedicated receptionist schedules new and return appointments	Suite check-in staff handle inbound telephones, scheduling	Shared telephone scheduler/messages in suite configuration	Central telephone scheduler/messages
RN schedules procedures/referrals	Central referral processing	Central referral processing	RN schedules procedures/referrals	Central referral processing
Central medical records without courier service	Central medical records without courier service	Medical records managed by suite check-in/check-out/medical records staff	Central medical records with courier service	Central medical records with courier service
Central check-in	Central check-in	Suite check-in staff	Suite check-in	Central check-in
Central check-out	Check-out performed by dedicated receptionist	Suite check-out (Check-in/check-out/medical records performed by same staff)	Suite check-out	Central check-out

spends a significant portion of time managing inbound telephone calls from patients involving prescription refills, test results reporting, nurse triage/advice, referral processing and scheduling procedures. The medical assistant is assigned to the physician exclusively and is responsible for rooming patients, conducting vitals and ensuring the rooms are stocked for a three exam room area. Due to the facility layout and the proximity of medical records to the patient check-in area, the medical assistant also provides courier service for medical records, frequently picking up charts from medical records and delivering them to the doctor's nurse.

PRIMARY CARE B

At the Primary Care B site, each physician has been delegated either a registered nurse or a licensed practical nurse and a dedicated receptionist. The dedicated receptionist is responsible for answering telephones, taking written telephone messages for the physician and nurse, ordering medical records (electronically), scheduling patient appointments, picking up medical records that have been pulled by medical records personnel and performing patient check-out functions, such as scheduling return appointments. The nurse is responsible for rooming patients and handling the telephone messages from patients. Referral processing is centralized, with the nurses providing the information electronically to the referral processing specialist. Patient check-in and medical records are centralized.

PRIMARY CARE C

At this primary care site, physicians are located in two-physician suites throughout the building. Each two-physician practice site has been delegated two nursing staff (LPN and MA combination) and three administrative/front office support staff. The clinical support staff rooms patients and responds to patient telephone inquiries. The three administrative support staff share the following functions: telephone messaging and patient scheduling, patient check-in, patient check-out and medical records filing and retrieval (medical records is decentralized). Referral processing has been centralized, with nursing staff providing the information on a form and faxing the form to a central referral processing coordinator.

PRIMARY CARE D

The fourth practice involves five physicians located in contiguous space. Each physician has his/her own registered nurse, and a medical assistant is assigned as a float to assist the nurses as needed. The nurses are responsible for rooming patients, handling patient telephone inquiries, scheduling procedures/referrals and scheduling some return patient appointments. Central telephone operators take telephone messages and schedule patient appointments. The telephone messages are electronically transmitted to central medical records; medical records staff then pull the chart and deliver both the chart and the message to the nurse on a continuous basis throughout the day. In this medical practice, patient check-in and patient check-out staff are shared among each five-physician group.

PRIMARY CARE E

The fifth and last practice in our example of practice models involves six physicians co-located in contiguous space. One medical assistant is assigned to two physicians (managing six exam rooms). Referral processing is centralized, with the medical assistant providing the information needed to correspond with the health plans. Central telephone operators take telephone messages for a central nurse triage unit, ordering the chart electronically, with the note and chart delivered to the nurse triage unit at the same time. The telephone operators also schedule patient appointments. Nurse triage staff handle the inbound patient telephone inquiries and dispense nurse advice. The nurses also have electronic access to radiology and clinical laboratory results. The majority of prescription refills are handled via pharmacy fax to medical records, with medical records staff pulling charts and delivering the request and chart to nurse triage staff at systematic time periods throughout the day. Patient check-in and patient check-out functions are provided centrally.

On a per FTE physician basis, the staffing patterns and staffing costs will be quite different, depending on the practice model that has been embraced. Primary Care Practice A, for example, will report a high clinical support staff per FTE physician since each physician has been delegated a nurse and a medical assistant. Primary Care Practice B will reflect higher levels of reception staff per FTE physician since each physician has been delegated his/her own receptionist to manage telephones, schedule appointments and to handle patient check-out.

A key question is "Which of these models is more efficient?" The answer is that it is dependent upon the physicians' workload, the facility layout, the technology, the patient scheduling methods, the workload of individual staff performing their current processes and other similar medical practice-specific factors. While there is no one "right way" to staff a medical practice, the staff rightsizing process takes these factors into account in the development of appropriate staffing models and staffing organization for the medical practice. Via the rightsizing process, each of these practice models can be reviewed to determine if they are optimal for a particular medical group.

AN IDEAL PEDIATRIC PRACTICE MODEL

Recognizing that internal medical practice-specific factors may present limitations, an ideal pediatric practice might involve assigning two physicians and one midlevel provider with one nurse and two medical assistants. Two of these configurations would be co-located into one practice suite.

The following assumptions are made as this model is more fully explored:

1. Provider workweek = 4.5 days;
2. Patient volume per provider = 32 patients per day; total = 145 patients per day;
3. Exam rooms = 12 to 15;
4. Medical records are maintained in the practice suite;
5. Pre-registration is performed centrally (not at suite level), involving registration and insurance verification;
6. The volume of referrals/testing/imaging is relatively low;
7. Systems support is available to maximize patient flow and streamline business processes.

TABLE 5.2 ■ Ideal Pediatric Staffing Model

	Check-in/Check-out/Referrals	2.00 FTE
	Medical Records	1.00 FTE
	Telephone Nurse Triage (LPN)	2.00 FTE
	Patient Scheduling	2.00 FTE
	Clinical Support (RN)	2.00 FTE
	Medical Assistants	4.00 FTE
	Total Staff FTE	**13.00 FTE**

TABLE 5.3 ■ Benchmark Comparison of Ideal Pediatric Staffing Model

Staff Title	Ideal Pediatric Per FTE Physician	MGMA Median	Ideal Pediatric Per FTE Provider	MGMA Median
Medical Receptionist Scheduling, Check-in, Check-out, Referrals	1.00	.97	.67	.78
Medical Records	.25	.35	.17	.25
Registered Nurses	.50	.57	.33	.39
Licensed Practical Nurse	.50	.27	.33	.42
Medical Assistants	1.00	.83	.67	.64
Total Staff	3.25	2.73	2.17	2.25

MGMA *Cost Survey: 2001 Report Based on 2000 Data*, Pediatrics, Median

Note: Total for MGMA data are from single specialty, pediatrics medical groups (not hospital owned). The total staff median was computed from the survey database and is not published in the survey report.

Note: This model assumes 2.00 FTE RN for back office support and 2.00 FTE LPN for nurse triage, however actual skill mix will be dependent upon scope of services performed.

Based upon the above assumptions, this staffing model would approximate MGMA median levels as shown in Table 5.3.

In summary, the front office and clinical support staff required for a particular practice is highly dependent upon the practice model that is adopted. Better performing medical practices adopt practice models that optimize not only the patient flow process but also staffing levels and staffing deployment.

■ PATIENT SCHEDULING

Differences in staffing support volumes and skill mix are also due to the type of patient scheduling model that is employed. For example, if a physician has adopted a sophisticated scheduling system, such as modified wave scheduling or advanced access scheduling, then the scheduling staff is highly engaged in bringing patients into the practice and optimizing the efficiency of the physician.

An example of the impact of patient scheduling on staffing is provided in Table 5.4 below. The data reflect the number of patients scheduled and the total number of hours from when the first patient is scheduled to when the last patient is scheduled during the day for five family practice physicians who have similar practices, including similar new-to-return patient ratios, similar volume of physicals, etc. During this particular week, there was high variability in average patients per scheduled hour of time. While some of this variability may be due to physician variation in practice style, the data suggest that there may be opportunities to enhance patient scheduling to improve physician efficiency. Large blocks of time during the day that are not scheduled efficiently will impact the ability of the physician to optimize efficiency, productivity and revenue.

TABLE 5.4 ■ Average Patients per Scheduled Hour per Physician

Physician	Monday	Tuesday	Wednesday	Thursday	Friday	Average Patients/ Scheduled Hour
Dr. A						
Patients	19	16	21	Not in	25	**5.14**
Scheduled Hours	4.5	3.0	5.25	clinic	3.0	
Dr. B						
Patients	24	24	23	Not in	21	**3.09**
Scheduled Hours	7.25	8.25	8.25	clinic	6.0	
Dr. C						
Patients	18	13	21	Not in	27	**3.40**
Scheduled Hours	7.0	2.75	7.0	clinic	6.5	
Dr. D						
Patients	23	Not in	26	21	19	**3.04**
Scheduled Hours	7.5	clinic	7.75	7.0	7.0	
Dr. E						
Patients	30	34	24	31	26	**3.74**
Scheduled Hours	7.0	8.25	7.25	8.0	8.25	

In the above example, the clinical staff support provided to each of the physicians in the practice includes both a registered nurse and a medical assistant. There would appear to be a significant amount of idle time during the day for some of these staff when patients are not seen. In this example, staffing utilization could be optimized with reductions in variability in how patients are scheduled throughout the day. If the patient scheduling process does not change, then adopting a group practice focus toward clinical staffing should be explored, consistent with the variability in patient volume per scheduled hour.

■ PRACTICE FACILITY

Space may be a limiting factor in a medical practice's ability to optimize staffing levels. An examination of the role facility design plays in enhancing productivity of the organization reveals variation among better performing medical practices and other practices. Better performing medical groups understand the importance of facility design in minimizing travel time by physicians in the practice and in optimizing exam room space to minimize wasted or unproductive time for the physician. Some examples of the impact of the practice facility on rightsizing staff are provided below.

1. PEDIATRIC PRACTICE A

Pediatric Practice A consists of 20 general and specialty pediatric practices located within a large practice facility that has been configured to permit physicians to practice in either their own office suite or in a two-physician suite arrangement, each with their own reception area. No common space has been delegated to medical records, thus each practice area maintains its own medical records.

Staffing Impact

The front-office staff will be replicated throughout the building at each of the practice sites, thereby limiting the ability to rightsize this staff based upon workload as measured by patient visit volume. Staff will be required in each area to maintain medical records. Finally, it will not be possible to rightsize clinical support staff due to the requirement for a one-to-one relationship with the physicians practicing in their own office suite.

2. Multispecialty Practice B

Multispecialty Practice B consists of eight physicians located in a moderately sized medical office building. Each physician has been assigned his/her own area in the building that consists of a nurse's station and three exam rooms. Due to the configuration of the building, the clinical space for each physician is essentially organized in separate hallways throughout the building. It is not possible for nursing staff, for example, to have visual contact with a hallway other than the one in which they are stationed.

Staffing Impact:

In this example, the practice may be able to optimize front office staffing, as the size of the physician group would suggest a central model for patient check-in and check-out functions. Clinical office support, however, probably will not be rightsized, as separate nursing stations per physician will impact the ability to provide for cross coverage by nursing staff to assist physicians in a more efficient staffing model.

TECHNOLOGY

Information technology and/or the ability of the practice to leverage technology may limit the ability of a practice to rightsize staff. If the medical practice has an electronic medical record, this, too, will impact the flow of staff in the practice. For example, with electronic medical records, the medical records personnel are not involved in chart retrieval and courier functions but instead spend time ensuring closed-loop processes for document scanning, patient notes, etc. Some examples of the impact of technology on staff rightsizing follow:

1. Medical Practice A

This particular practice has a practice management software system that does not permit the co-payment to be posted prior to the patient visit. Consequently, collection of co-payments is conducted at the time of patient check-out. This limits the ability of the practice to minimize check-out functions or eliminate them altogether, a trend seen in many practices today.

2. MEDICAL PRACTICE B

This practice is not able to use its technology to "arrive" the patient. That is, rather than notifying the clinical support area of patient arrival via the use of technology (examples of this include automated arrival on the scheduling system, printing of charge tickets and/or labels in the back office as notification of patient arrival, use of digital pagers or other electronic means), the medical record continues to be used as a "queue" to the medical assistant that the patient has arrived.

Staffing inefficiency is thus inherent in this patient arrival process:

- The front office staff maintains the medical record prior to appointment rather than the clinical support staff, thus preparation for the patient visit by clinical staff to ensure that the medical record is up-to-date and to anticipate needs for the visit is not performed;
- The front office employees leave their work station to take the medical record to the clinical area; and
- The medical assistants periodically interrupt their work to see if the medical record has been delivered.

In addition to these internal medical practice-specific factors to be considered when rightsizing, environmental and market factors may also impact rightsizing efforts for a medical group. Some examples of this follow.

PATIENT ACCEPTANCE OF TECHNOLOGY

The ability of a practice to implement telephony products may impact the number of staff needed in the medical practice. An automated attendant, for example, permits many practices to reduce staffing levels for telephone operators; however, an automated attendant may or may not be viewed as an acceptable access method by patients. As another example, some telephony products permit patients to access their test results via dial-up to the practice. While this reduces inbound telephone volume and minimizes direct staff interaction with the patient, the acceptability of this approach may be precluded by market demand. Finally, some practices permit patients to schedule their appointments via a secure Web site, a procedure that could lead to a reduction in the number of staff required for patient scheduling. The use of this patient scheduling method, however, is dependent upon the level to which patients embrace this process and technology.

GEOGRAPHIC DESIGNATION OF THE PRACTICE

The geographic designation of the practice also may impact the staff rightsizing process. A number of studies have found that those physicians practicing in higher population density areas tend to see less patient visits than their rural physician counterparts. Since staff cost is a step-fixed cost to the practice, higher patient volumes could require higher staffing levels for practices, based on their geographic designation.

Level of Managed Care and Capitation

Practices with high levels of managed care penetration may exhibit the need for different staffing work functions. For example, staff may be involved in more administrative paperwork associated with pre-authorization, referral management, multiple formularies and laboratories and other similar work than those without multiple health plan requirements. Similarly, practices with high capitation levels may invest in nurse triage units more aggressively in order to ensure patient access and minimize unnecessary emergency room or clinic visits. In addition, practices that are involved in global capitation arrangements may exhibit different practice scope and service offerings to patients, necessitating a different staffing skill mix. Thus, it is important to recognize these types of market-related factors when determining if the staff is rightsized in a medical practice.

A Systematic Approach to Rightsizing the Medical Practice

CHAPTER 6

Conducting a systematic approach to rightsizing staff in the medical practice involves five discrete steps:

Step 1: **Benchmark the Current State**
Question to Resolve: Does the data suggest areas of opportunity?

Step 2: **Analyze Current Productivity**
Question to Resolve: How productive are the employees?

Step 3: **Analyze Current Practice Model**
Question to Resolve: Should a change in practice model be explored?

Step 4: **Analyze Process Performance**
Question to Resolve: Are key work processes encumbered?

Step 5: **Take Action**
Question to Resolve: What action should be taken?

In *Step 1-Benchmark the Current State,* benchmarking is used to determine whether or not there are opportunities for change or improvement that are suggested by the data. This allows medical practice executives to focus on critical areas within the practice and ask key questions such as:

1. Does the practice have the right number of staff?
2. Does it have the right mix of staff?
3. Are staffing expenditures appropriate?
4. Is the staff contributing to practice profitability?
5. Are there clear areas of opportunity?

It is important to remember that, as addressed earlier, there may be a number of internal practice-specific limiting factors that need to be taken into account, but benchmarking is the first step to permit a focus on the current staffing model of the practice and to start asking questions about staffing workload and productivity.

Step 2-Analyze Current Productivity involves analyzing the current productivity of employees in the practice. This permits an understanding of the productivity of employees when they perform critical business functions. Productivity workload ranges that are developed by the practice are used to understand where the practice has opportunity for change or improvement. The questions that are asked in this step include:

1. What are the staffing utilization levels for critical work processes?
2. Is more or less support staff needed to perform these functions if the current work process is not changed?
3. What are the expected performance outcomes? Have they been met?

In *Step 3-Analyze Current Practice Model,* the current practice model and staffing model are analyzed to determine whether changes to the model could facilitate staff rightsizing and enhance productivity, efficiency and profitability. Key questions to address in this step are:

1. What type of practice model has been embraced?
2. What is the purpose of the current practice model?
3. Is there another practice model that could enhance efficiency and service?
4. Is the facility presenting a limitation for efficient practice?
5. Is the medical practice taking advantage of economies of scale?
6. What duties have been delegated to staff?
7. To what extent have specific functions been shared or distributed?
8. Who are the key parties to involve in model discussions?

Step 4-Analyze Specific Work Processes involves analyzing process performance. It is important to understand that the core business processes and systems actually produce the costs, not staff per se. For practices that want to embrace a strategy that is different from simply "managing costs," it is important to look at the performance of **processes.**[10] It is not the staff that causes the cost, it is the systems and processes that the staff is asked to perform that dictate the volume and type of staff required for the process. Step 4 involves focusing on the activities and processes, not simply costs.

Questions to address as part of Step 4 are:

1. What is the goal of this particular process?
2. What are the boundaries of the process?
3. What is the current process?
4. What are the current process measures?
5. Is there a better way to perform this process?

In the final step, *Step 5-Take Action,* medical practices take action to achieve desired change. "Rightsizing only provides you with data. If the data aren't used to make good business decisions to drive important change efforts and change current staffing strategies, rightsizing will be of little value."[11]

---

[10]Mozena JP, Emerick CE, Black SC. Stop Managing Costs: Designing Health Care Organizations Around Core Business Systems. Milwaukee: ASQ Quality Press; 1999.

[11]Adapted from Brown MG. Keeping Score: Using the Right Metrics to Drive World-Class Performance. New York: Quality Resources; 1996.

STEP 1: BENCHMARK THE CURRENT STATE

Benchmarking facilitates an understanding of the current staffing volumes and skill mix of staff in the medical practice and compares this with: (1) peer practices and (2) practices that are considered "better performing" medical groups (those that have achieved higher levels of performance and better financial results) to learn what other groups have done to achieve their results. With national data collected by the Medical Group Management Association, medical practice executives are able to analyze real world information and examine what happens when practices have different staffing levels.

Benchmarking is a very simple activity. It is basically setting goals knowing what others are doing. The concept of benchmarking has to do with looking at relationships and helping practices understand where they are in relation to the performance of others. Benchmarking data available today move beyond simply knowledge about the performance of the general population of medical practices. Data are now available on better performing medical practices that permit an examination of a specific group of practices to learn what they are doing differently that permits them to achieve higher performance levels. Examining these better performing practices permits medical practice executives to import ideas and/or model activity from better performing practices. Finally, it is important to understand that benchmarking is an ongoing process; it is not just a one time event.

Why Benchmark?

Benchmarking permits medical practices to accomplish five important goals. First, benchmarking facilitates understanding of the performance of key processes and performance outcomes. This has to do with the concept of measurement. With measurement, medical practice executives are able to better understand the performance of their medical practices.

Secondly, benchmarking permits health care leaders to view the performance of their own practices over time. One of the most important concepts of benchmarking is to understand whether or not performance is improving or deteriorating. If a decision is made to change staffing levels or the staffing model, what results are expected? A time series benchmark—a before measure and an after measure—is needed that reflects the performance of the practice before the intervention so that medical practice executives are able to evaluate the positive or perhaps even the negative aspects of that intervention.

FIGURE 6.1 ■ Why Benchmark?

> Benchmarking permits medical practices to accomplish five important goals:
> 1. Facilitates understanding of key processes and performance outcomes;
> 2. Permits health care leaders to view the performance of their own practices over time;
> 3. Permits comparison of measurements against peer groups;
> 4. Provides an opportunity to analyze the processes of others to understand what they do differently; and
> 5. Convinces others of the need for change.

Third, benchmarking permits comparison of measurements against peer groups. These include average comparisons as well as comparisons with organizations that exhibit higher levels of performance—organizations that are considered better performing medical practices. Another important goal of benchmarking is that it provides an opportunity to analyze the processes of others to understand what they do differently. Some organizations benchmark their activity to organizations outside of their own industry to determine if there are innovative opportunities that have not been considered and to better understand how they want to do business. For example, a medical practice executive may want to examine the processing of accounts in the banking industry to facilitate better understanding of the physician billing process or accounts payable process or perhaps to examine the hotel industry to learn of opportunities to enhance patient satisfaction. Medical practice executives may want to look at many other industries that are not involved in health care, and may apply innovative, creative ideas learned to their own medical practices (and in the process perhaps even become a "best practice" for others to emulate).

The final goal of benchmarking is to convince others of the need for change. This is basically overcoming "mural dyslexia," or the inability of an individual or a group of individuals to read the handwriting on the wall. At times, health care leaders find themselves in positions where they need to convince administrators, physicians, midlevel providers, managers, supervisors, support staff and others that change is needed. Benchmarking the current state of the medical practice against other practices can often assist in moving the organization forward or better positioning the organization to achieve its strategic goals.

THE TEN-STEP BENCHMARKING PROCESS

The 10-step benchmarking process is reflected in Figure 6.2. It involves establishing objectives, identifying performance indices and benchmarking sources, collecting data, performing a gap analysis, finding out why a practice's information differs from the benchmark and communicating the findings among physicians and staff. It consists of developing action plans, initiating change and reassessing the practice's objectives. Benchmarking is an ongoing process. Once the process has been completed, it involves beginning the entire process yet again. The 10 benchmarking steps are continually repeated in the organization, allowing health care leaders to set objectives, measure performance

FIGURE 6.2 ■ The 10-Step Benchmarking Process

1. Establish practice objectives
2. Identify performance indices (what to measure)
3. Identify benchmark sources available
4. Collect data
5. Perform data comparison and GAP analysis
6. Communicate findings
7. Develop action and assessment plans
8. Implement plans and monitor progress
9. Assess practice objectives, evaluate benchmark standards, recalibrate measurement
10. REPEAT

and then move on and do this again and again in order to continually enhance and improve the organization.

Benchmarking Metrics

There are two major types of metrics available for benchmarking purposes: (1) peer performance measures and (2) "better performing" medical practice measures. Better performing practices are organizations that have higher levels of performance. Data are available at median levels, as well as by quartiles in order to provide reference for benchmarking one's own medical group. Typically, medical practices begin the benchmarking analysis using median data in comparison to their peers to determine initial areas of opportunity.

FIGURE 6.3 ■ Two Types of Benchmarking Metrics

1. Peer Performance Measures
2. Better Performing Medical Practice Measures

The Median Performance Measure: A median is a statistic that represents the "mid-point" of reported data. Median benchmarks for staffing the medical practice are published in the MGMA *Cost Survey Report*. The MGMA *Cost Survey* has been conducted for the past 50 years. With more than 1,000 organizations participating in the survey, this survey represents a robust database for benchmarking analysis.

Better Performing Practices Median: Published since 1999, the MGMA *Performance and Practices of Successful Medical Groups Report* provides median data for better performing medical groups. Better performing medical groups are those groups selected based on quantitative performance thresholds that resulted in higher levels of financial success or "more profit to the bottom line." Once better performers were identified, researchers, consultants and MGMA staff examined what these practices were doing that served to distinguish their higher levels of performance so that others might learn from their success.

The benchmarks for family practice are provided in Table 6.1. In this table, staffing benchmark data are provided at the median level for single specialty family practice groups. For purposes of benchmark comparisons, the data are available for two types of family practices: those owned by hospitals or integrated delivery systems (IDS) and those that are not owned by hospitals or integrated delivery systems. Hospital or integrated delivery system ownership has some very definitive effects on staffing patterns; many of the staff positions typically reported by medical practices either may reside in the parent hospital or are provided elsewhere in the system. The data reflected in Table 6.1 are standardized on a per full-time equivalent (FTE) physician basis. The median or midpoint of the staffing is 4.67 support staff per FTE physician for family practice single specialty groups that are not hospital or IDS owned, and 4.47 FTE support staff per FTE physician for those family practice groups that are hospital- or IDS-owned. Better performing family practice groups have a median of 5.25 support staff per FTE physician.

Graph 6.1 reflects a histogram or simply a distribution of differing levels of staff for family practice groups that are not hospital- or IDS-owned. The midpoint of 4.67 staff occurs almost at the same point as the mean. A classic bell-shaped curve is demonstrated; however it should be noted that the variance between practices is substantial. Some practices have as

TABLE 6.1 ■ Staffing for Family Practice Single Specialty Groups, by Ownership, per FTE Physician

	\multicolumn{4}{c}{Not Hospital / IDS-Owned}	\multicolumn{4}{c}{Hospital / IDS-Owned}
	Count	25th %tile	Median	75th %tile	Count	25th %tile	Median	75th %tile
General administrative FTE	49	0.17	0.24	0.32	15	0.10	0.18	0.32
Business office FTE	53	0.55	0.80	1.07	32	0.32	0.50	1.61
Managed care administrative FTE	16	0.09	0.16	0.25	7	*	*	*
Information technology FTE	6	*	*	*	3	*	*	*
Housekeeping, maintenance, security FTE	13	0.08	0.14	0.33	2	*	*	*
Medical receptionists FTE	51	0.68	1.00	1.25	18	0.76	1.13	1.49
Medical secretaries, transcribers FTE	37	0.20	0.34	0.56	20	0.22	0.33	0.43
Medical records FTE	40	0.27	0.43	0.65	14	0.22	0.34	0.58
Other administrative support FTE	13	0.11	0.13	0.17	16	0.16	1.08	2.00
Registered nurses FTE	41	0.23	0.44	0.77	22	0.29	0.50	0.89
Licensed practical nurses FTE	46	0.25	0.40	0.79	30	0.39	0.95	1.45
Medical assistants, nurse's aides FTE	44	0.40	0.76	1.09	24	0.23	0.45	0.82
Clinical laboratory FTE	36	0.24	0.34	0.51	13	0.17	0.30	0.39
Radiology and imaging FTE	30	0.14	0.21	0.29	11	0.14	0.20	0.33
Other medical support services FTE	8	*	*	*	3	*	*	*
Total contracted support staff FTE	21	0.09	0.23	0.43	7	*	*	*
Total support staff FTE	56	4.08	4.67	5.45	40	3.79	4.47	5.28

Total FTE Support Staff per FTE Physician
Family Practice (Not Hospital / IDS-Owned)

Std. Dev = 1.37
Mean = 4.89
N = 55.00

Total Support Staff per FTE Physician

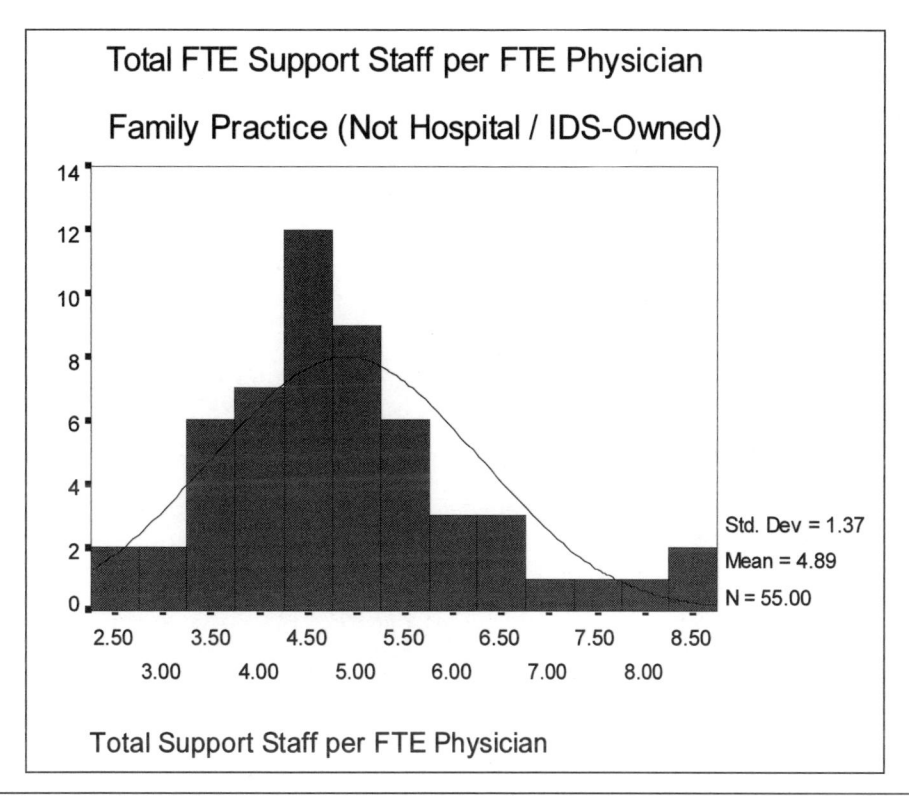

GRAPH 6.1 ■ Histogram: Staffing for Family Practice Single Specialty Groups (Not Hospital/IDS-Owned)

few as 2.50 staff per physician, and some practices have 8.50 staff per physician. This indicates that there is a variation in staffing patterns among these family practice medical groups.

We will now explore the data in greater depth to begin to understand the impact of staffing levels on the medical practice.

Graph 6.2 is a scatter plot. A scatter plot demonstrates where the results lie compared across two different axes. The x-axis or horizontal axis reflects total FTE support staff per FTE physician, while the y-axis or vertical axis reflects total medical revenue per FTE physician. For example, the practice that had 8.50 employees per doctor also happened to report one of the highest levels of total medical revenue per FTE physician.

A regression line is also demonstrated on this graph. The regression line permits the opportunity to look at the path of center of the data so that conclusions may be drawn from the relationship between the total FTE support staff and total medical revenue (the x-axis and y-axis, respectively). As demonstrated, the regression line is vertical, thus there is a relationship between having more staff and having more revenue. In fact there is an inferential statistic called an R^2 that demonstrates the relationship of these two values. The R^2 in this instance is .4769, meaning that approximately 48 percent of the change in medical revenue can be attributed to the increased number of staff. This supports the belief that the more staff a practice has, the greater the opportunity for production and the greater the opportunity for revenue generation.

Graph 6.3 is constructed to permit us to learn the consequence of having these employees. The vertical axis reflects total operating cost per FTE physician, while the horizontal axis

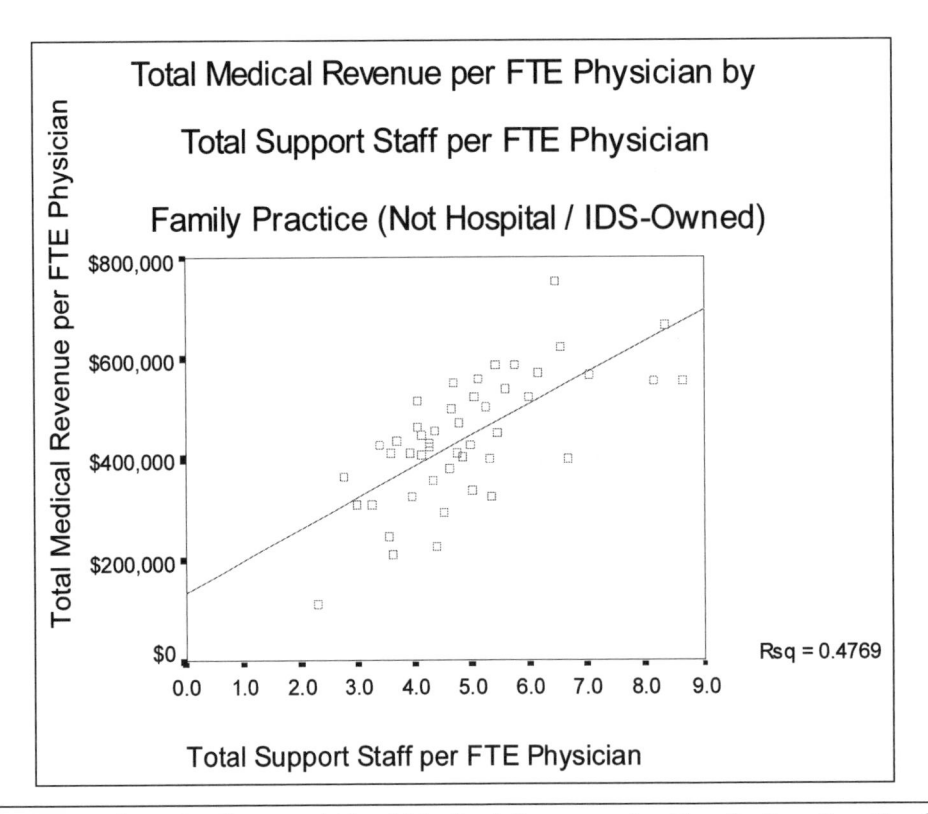

GRAPH 6.2 ■ Scatterplot: Staffing and Total Medical Revenue for Family Practice Single Specialty Groups (Not Hospital/IDS-Owned)

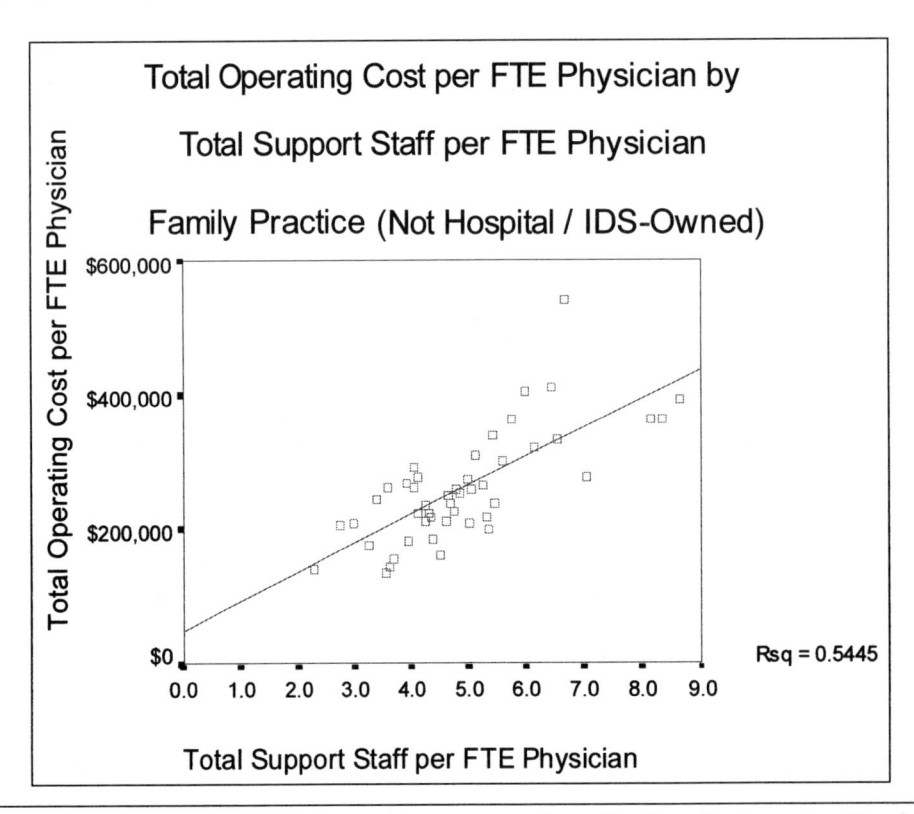

GRAPH 6.3 ■ Scatterplot: Staffing and Total Operating Cost for Family Practice Single Specialty Groups (Not Hospital/IDS-Owned)

is the same total FTE support staff per FTE physician as reported in the earlier graphs. This graph demonstrates that not only does the cost of practice increase with more staff, but there is even a stronger relationship of having more staff to having higher cost. In this case 54 percent of the change in total operating cost is a result of the change in total support staff per FTE physician.

The last scatter plot (Graph 6.4) is the telltale activity that demonstrates the relationship between total FTE support staff and revenue after operating cost or the net benefit to the practice. Revenue after operating cost in a partnership or professional corporation is the revenue that is distributed to the physician owners either as compensation, as benefits or as retained earnings. This scatter diagram demonstrates that there is a positive relationship between total FTE support staff and revenue after operating costs, albeit a weak one (9 percent of the change in revenue after operating cost per FTE physician is attributed to total support staff per FTE physician).

This data suggest that practices with higher ratios of staff per FTE physician have higher revenues, expenses go up as staffing ratios increase, and there is a positive, although weak relationship between higher levels of staff to increases in revenue after operating cost. **It suggests that better performing practices have increased profitability not as a result of having more staff but of having the right staff.**

These are the first benchmarks to use to obtain an understanding of how others staff their medical practices, but they further beg the question of what these organizations are doing differently in order to achieve higher levels of performance. An examination of medical practices that have higher levels of revenue after operating cost and lower cost per

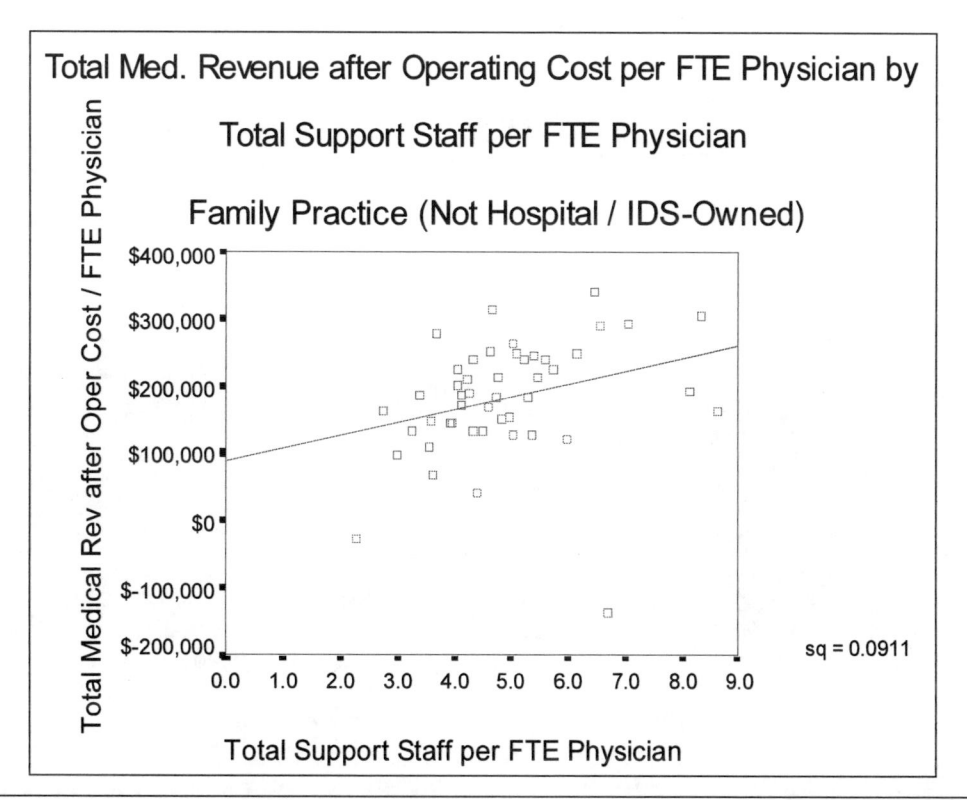

GRAPH 6.4 ■ Scatterplot: Staffing and Total Revenue After Operating Cost for Family Practice Single Specialty Groups (Not Hospital/IDS-Owned)

procedure reveals that these better performing practices have lower costs, higher revenues, higher physician compensation and benefit levels, and enhanced productivity. And we also see that one of the reasons for enhanced productivity is a slightly different concentration of staff. Graph 6.5 demonstrates that these practices do, indeed, generate higher revenue. In addition, Graph 6.6 shows that these practices reflect a slightly higher staff cost per FTE physician. (Note: The higher cost per physician may be due to the higher volume of staff per FTE physician, higher wage rates, and/or a different skill mix of staff.)

The important question is: *What are these practices doing differently relative to staffing strategies that may help explain their success?* Medical practice executives and physicians interviewed in these organizations indicate that they place a strong emphasis on improving their key revenue processes. "They do the right things, and they do them right." They systematically perform pre-visit functions, including verifying insurance and checking for pre-authorization for services. They focus attention on billing and collection processes, maximizing their time-of-service payments. They emphasize correct coding and compliance with appropriate regulations and health plan requirements. They devote a substantial amount of energy to ensuring a "clean claim" and to actively managing their contracts. Physicians practice efficiently by dictating throughout the day rather than delaying work, and they maximize their clinical time. Physicians delegate appropriately to nurses and other staff in the practice, with all organizational members focused on optimizing productivity

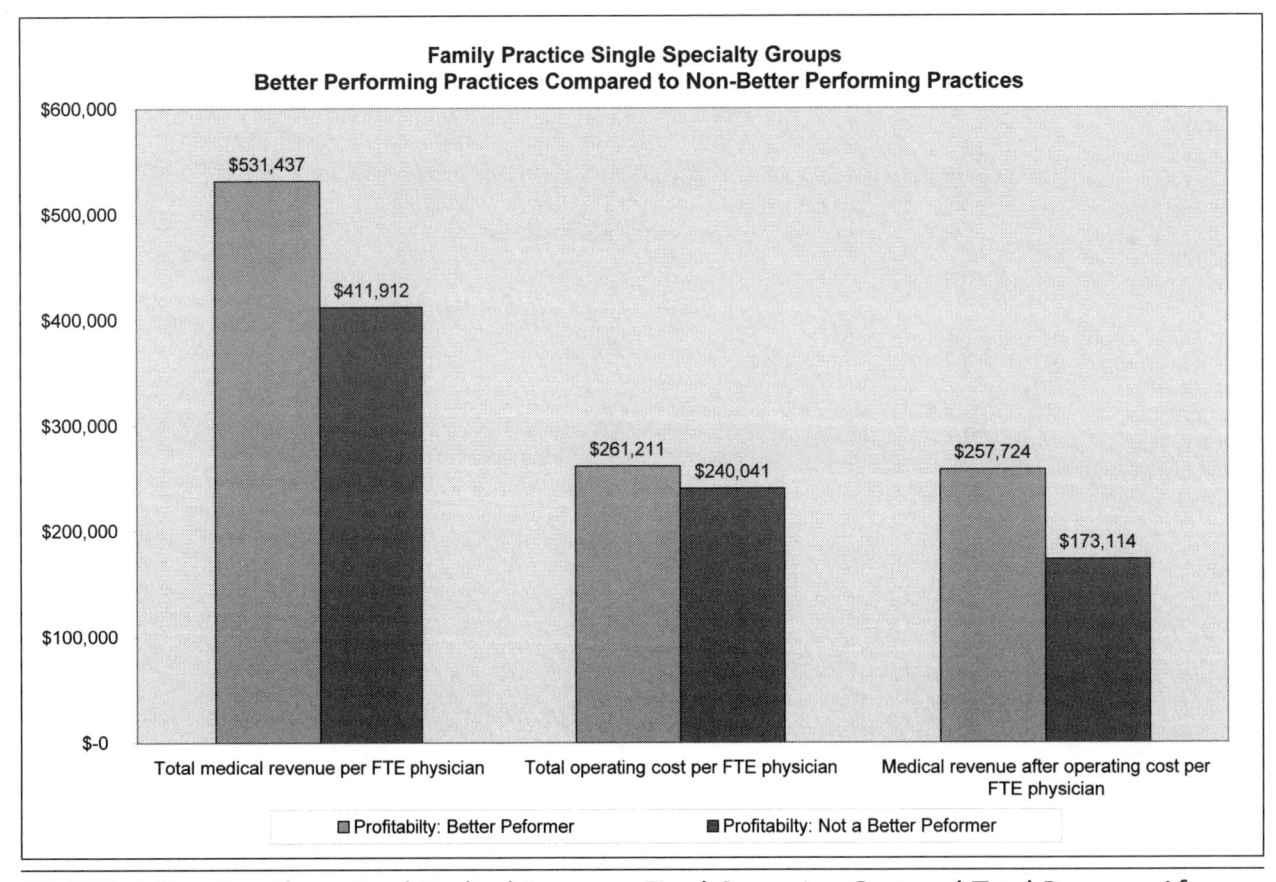

GRAPH 6.5 ■ Bar Chart: Total Medical Revenue, Total Operating Cost and Total Revenue After Operating Cost per FTE Physician, Family Practice Single Specialty Groups (Better Performing Practices Compared to Not Better Performing Practices)

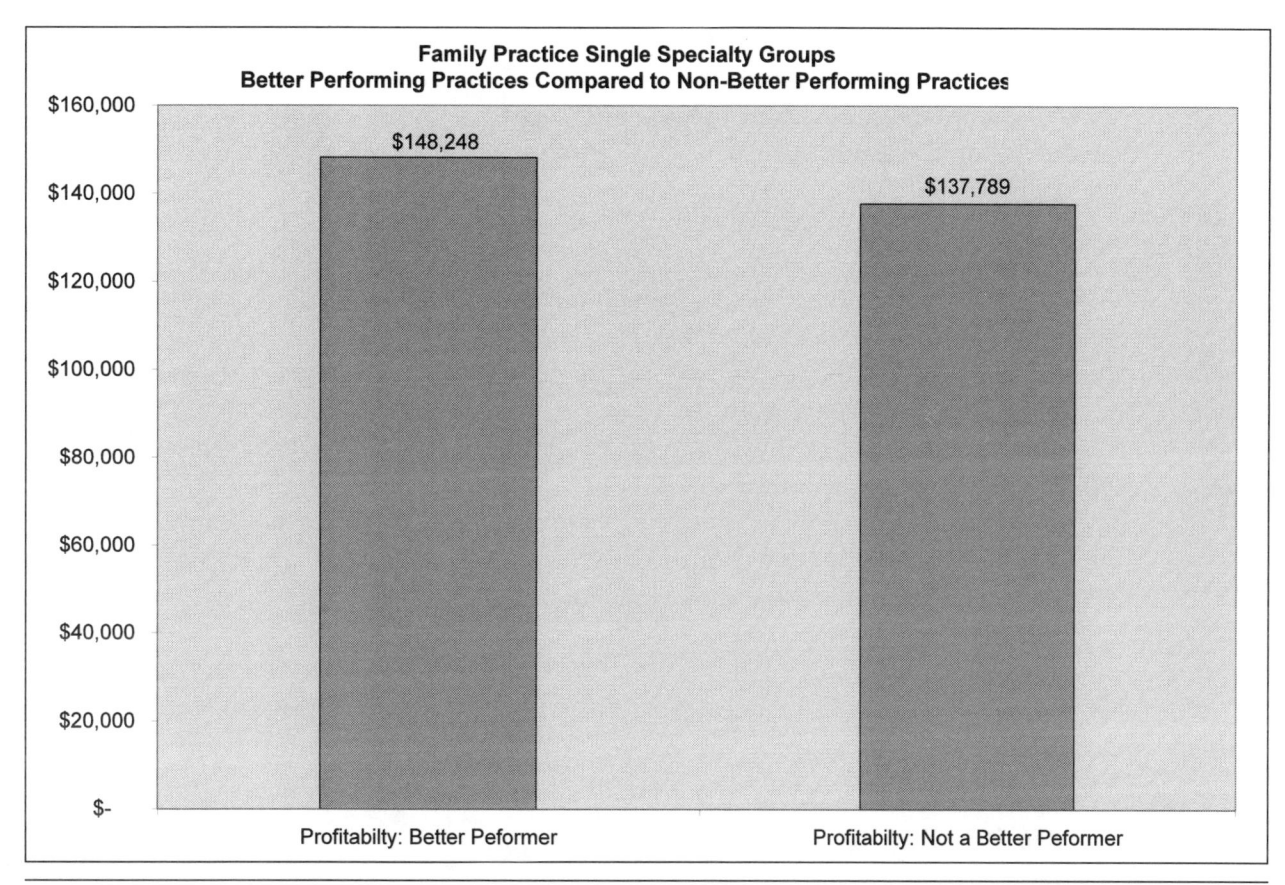

GRAPH 6.6 ■ Bar Chart: Total Support Staff Cost per FTE Physician, Family Practice Single Specialty Groups (Better Performing Practices Compared to Not Better Performing Practices)

and efficiency. Better performing medical groups focus on managing costs, including lowering per unit costs, such as maximizing facility utilization to lower the cost of a patient visit, managing supplies and other overhead expenditures.

Examining these practices further, we found that the incentives provided in the physician compensation programs of better performing medical groups reward productivity. Anecdotally through interviews, these organizations state that they apply substantial resources to retaining staff and training the staff that they have in order to enhance practice productivity and efficiency and to achieve performance outcomes. These practices recognize the high cost of staff turnover, not only in recruitment and training costs but in lost productivity and intellectual capital for the practice; and they take active steps to retain good employees. A recurring comment that better performing practices make is that they focus on reimbursing and rewarding staff for their hard work.

Benchmarking and Staff Rightsizing

When benchmarking for staff rightsizing, a number of different measures should be utilized and collectively assessed to determine whether there is opportunity to rightsize the medical practice. Benchmarking can be conducted internally, comparing data among practice sites within the medical group, as well as externally, comparing this data with external benchmarks of practices of similar specialty, size, or ownership and/or comparing it with better performing medical practices.

Six quantitative measures are typically used to assess staffing levels and perform benchmarking comparison:

1. Staff FTE per FTE Physician, per FTE Clinical Equivalent Physician, and/or per FTE Provider

This measure compares overall staffing levels on a per FTE basis. This is typically the first level of benchmarking, as it reflects staffing on a per FTE physician basis, and it permits analysis of overall levels of opportunity. In academic practices where physicians have clinical, research and academic responsibilities, or if physicians have substantial time devoted to administration, it is important to understand physician productivity and staffing levels calculated on a per Clinical Equivalent FTE (CFTE) basis. Typically the current actual physician productivity as measured by work relative value units is compared to median work relative value benchmark levels to calculate a CFTE equivalency measure. If, for example, CFTE levels are actually higher than FTE levels in a practice productivity of the physicians may warrant higher staffing levels.

For practices that have a high number of midlevel providers, analyzing the data on a per-FTE provider level as well as on a per-physician level is recommended. This will permit the medical practice to examine its staffing strategy in relation to total providers in the practice.

2. Staff FTE by Staff Category and by Job Classification Level per FTE Physician and/or per FTE Provider

This next level of benchmarking permits a comparison of staffing devoted to actual work functions within the medical practice. Data in Appendix III and Appendix IV delineate a number of staffing categories involving administrative and business functions, front office functions, clinical support functions and ancillary services, with detailed job classification levels reported in each of these categories. This level of staffing analysis permits identification of opportunity related to specific job functions performed in the practice as well as staffing skill mix. For example, a practice may elect to employ only registered nurses whereas its benchmark counterpart has a blend of registered nurses, licensed practical nurses and medical assistants.

3. Staff FTE per Various Outputs, such as Relative Value Units, Work Relative Value Units, Patients, Patient Visits

A comparison of staffing FTE to various outputs permits an understanding of variability in productivity among practices and the potential need for different infrastructures based on production levels. Staffing is a measure of work. Staffing per work relative value units and per number of patients are two common measures to compute to determine whether staffing on a quantitative performance output measure may suggest opportunities to right-size the practice. This type of analysis recognizes that staffing relates to the work activity that is performed.

4. Staff FTE per Various Inputs, such as Specialty, Facility Square Footage

As previously discussed, staffing levels will vary depending upon the specialty of the physicians, with primary care physicians requiring more staff on a per FTE basis than their surgical colleagues. In addition, the size of the practice facility will also impact the number of staff needed to perform various functions as patient flow, courier functions and other duties may be impacted by the size of the physical space. A staffing benchmarking analysis based on these types of inputs will assist practices in determining areas of rightsizing opportunity.

5. Staff Cost Per FTE Physician

A determination of staff cost per FTE physician permits identification of the variable cost levels associated with staffing levels and skill mix of staff. It should be noted, however, that a number of reasons could be attributed to a finding of higher staff cost per physician. Staffing levels could be higher, thus staffing cost on a per FTE physician basis would be expected to be higher. Alternatively, higher wages could be paid to the staff, also yielding higher cost on a per FTE basis. Finally, a different skill mix of staff, such as higher levels of registered nurses rather than medical assistants, could translate to higher staff cost on a per-physician FTE basis. In many cases, a combination of the above serve as the explanatory factor for a finding of higher staff cost. If a medical practice regularly incurs a significant overtime expense, this expense can be translated to an FTE equivalent level based on hours worked, and should be taken into account when analyzing staffing levels and staffing expenditures.

6. Staff Cost As a Percent of Total Medical Revenue

Of the six quantitative measures, staff cost as a percent of total medical revenue is particularly useful, because it addresses two important questions: 1) Does the practice have the right staff; and 2) Is the staff doing the right things? Data provided in Appendix III and Appendix IV permit analysis of staffing cost as a percent of total medical revenue at the level of staff category as well as at the job classification level.

Better performing practices typically have more staff than other practices and have higher staffing cost on a per FTE physician basis than other practices, yet have lower cost as a percent of total medical revenue than other practices. A conclusion drawn from the data is that better performing practices have the right staff doing the right things that are contributing to practice profitability.

When comparing staffing patterns of medical groups using the measure of staff cost as a percent of total medical revenue, however, it is also important to analyze the factors that contribute to total medical revenue. Important factors to analyze when reviewing revenue performance include:

- Payer mix;
- Specialty mix (practices that offer primary care services only would have a higher staffing cost as a percent of total medical revenue than practices that offer both primary and specialty services);
- Scope of services (practices that have on-site ancillary services may have a greater revenue-generating capability than those sites that do not have this added revenue stream);
- Physician productivity; and
- Billing and collection practices.

In summary, this first step in the staff rightsizing process is intended to permit examination of the medical practice's staffing in comparison to benchmarks of peer practices and better performing medical practices. Benchmarking allows medical practice executives to ask key questions regarding staffing levels and staffing deployment:

1. Does the practice have the right number of staff?
2. Does it have the right mix of staff?
3. Are staffing expenditures appropriate?
4. Is the staff contributing to practice profitability?
5. Are there clear areas of opportunity?

BENCHMARKING CASE STUDY

An example of the benchmarking process is presented in the form of a case study. Premier Multispecialty Group consists of seven physicians practicing in one location performing primary care services only. In Step 1-Benchmarking the Current State, its current staffing levels will be compared with national benchmarks.

To calculate staff FTE ratios per FTE physician, the practice administrator has reviewed each staff position and has identified the hours each staff member spends in various functions. Note that this goes beyond the job classification or title code of the staff member to reflect the time the employee actually spends on various tasks in the medical practice.

Six quantitative measures will be computed for Premier Multispecialty Group as part of the benchmarking comparison. These measures are used collectively to determine if there is opportunity to rightsize the practice and to suggest areas of process performance that warrant investigation.

TABLE 6.2 ■ Staff Time Devoted to Specific Tasks (embedded in text)

Number of Staff	Job Classification	Activity	Time Hours/Week
1	Practice Administrator	Manages practice	40
3	Registered Nurse	Clinical nursing	90
		Referral management	10
7	Licensed Practical Nurse	Clinical nursing	260
4	Medical Assistant	Clinical support/patient flow	110
		Reception/check-in	30
		Patient scheduling	20
4	Receptionists	Check-in/phones/check-out	160
1	Medical Records Clerk	Medical records filing/retrieval	40
3	Billing Staff	Billing and collections	120
3	Ancillary Staff	Clinical laboratory	80
		Radiology	40
26			1,000 hours

1. Staff FTE per Physician FTE

Normal workweek for this practice:	40 hours
Total FTE support staff:	1,000 hours/40 hours = 25.00 FTE staff
Total physicians:	7.00 FTE
Total FTE support staff per FTE physician:	25.00/7.00 = 3.57 FTE

Determination of the number of physicians in a practice may require close examination. For example, if the practice recognizes a 40-hour workweek, and a physician only works 30 hours each week, the physician would be a .75 FTE physician, not a 1.00 FTE physician. In addition, a physician who sees 22 patients per day and a physician who sees 38 patients a day may have different staffing needs; however both may be considered "full time" in the practice. In this case study we are assuming that all seven physicians are working full time in the practice (7.00 FTE physicians) and that they have similar workloads.

2. Staff FTE by Staff Categories and Job Classification Levels Per Physician FTE

Premier Multispecialty Group can now compare its current staffing categories and job classification levels to the normative benchmarks. This is depicted in Table 6.3 below. Note that the activity reported by the staff members was mapped to the benchmark definitions so that specific staffing categories can be compared. This permits the group to identify areas of opportunity and areas of focus for improvements to its staffing strategy.

At the level of staffing categories, it appears that there may be opportunity to rightsize staff in a number of areas for Premier Multispecialty Group. For example, the number of administrative and business staff is considerably lower than benchmark levels, as is the number of front office staff. The number of clinical support staff and ancillary staff, however, more closely approximate benchmark norms.

Table 6.4 provides a more detailed view of the staffing in Premier Multispecialty Group in comparison to the actual job classification levels of the employees. This permits an opportunity to review staffing skill mix as well as individual job classification levels that may be targeted for review in the rightsizing process.

At first glance, one might want to draw the conclusion that Premier Multispecialty Group is understaffed since the MGMA median benchmark reflects 5.00 FTE support staff per FTE physician, with Premier Multispecialty Group only reporting 3.57 FTE support staff per FTE physician. It should be noted, however, that the MGMA benchmarking data report staff for categories that are not reported by Premier Multispecialty Group. For example,

TABLE 6.3 ■ Benchmarking Staff Categories

Staff Category	Premier Total Staff FTE	Premier Per FTE Physician	MGMA Median
Administrative & Business Staff	4.00	.57	1.61
Front Office Staff	6.25	.89	1.06
Clinical Staff	11.75	1.68	1.75
Ancillary Service Staff	3.00	.43	.56
TOTAL	25.00	3.57	5.00

Source: Appendix III, Table 4d. Data derived from *MGMA Cost Survey: 2001 Report Based on 2000 Data,* Multispecialty Practices with Primary Care Only, Not Owned by Hospital or Integrated Delivery System.

TABLE 6.4 ■ Benchmarking Staff Classification Levels

Staff Title	Premier Total Staff FTE	Premier Per FTE Physician	MGMA Median
Administrative & Business Support Staff			
General administrative	1.00	.14	.25
Business office	3.00	.43	.71
Managed care	.00	.00	*
Information technology	.00	.00	.11
Housekeeping/maintenance/security	.00	.00	.14
Front Office & Clerical Staff			
Medical receptionists	5.25	.75	1.16
Medical secretaries/transcribers	.00	.00	.29
Medical records	1.00	.14	.31
Other administrative support	.00	.00	.18
Clinical Support Staff			
Registered nurses	2.50	.36	.44
Licensed practical nurses	6.50	.93	.50
Medical assistants, aides	2.75	.39	.74
Ancillary Staff			
Clinical laboratory	2.00	.29	.37
Radiology and imaging	1.00	.14	.23
Other medical support	.00	.00	.20
Total employed staff	**25.00**	**3.57**	**4.94**
Contracted support staff	.00	.00	.24
Total support staff	**25.00**	**3.57**	**5.00**

* Data not reported due to insufficient number of responses.

Source: Appendix III, Table 4a. Data derived from MGMA *Cost Survey: 2001 Report Based on 2000 Data*, Multispecialty Practices with Primary Care Only, Not Owned by Hospital or Integrated Delivery System.

medical transcription staff are included in the benchmarking source data; however, Premier Multispecialty Group outsources its transcription and thus does not report staffing levels for this work function.

This detailed level of analysis helps to define the categories and job classification levels of opportunity to be explored. For example, in the general support staff category, there may be opportunities in the area of business and administrative functions to rightsize the staff and to obtain higher performance outcomes. In the area of front office staff, the medical reception category is particularly low, suggesting opportunity to review work functions and tasks and to determine if the pre-visit, check-in, referral, collection of time-of-service payments, and other functions are performed at optimal levels. In the area of clinical support staff, the skill mix of staff at Premier Multispecialty Group differs from its benchmark counterparts, again prompting questions such as whether the nurses are performing nursing duties that require licensure and whether tasks have been delegated to staff consistent with their classification.

3. Staff FTE per Various Outputs, such as Relative Value Units, Work Relative Value Units, Patients, Patient Visits

A benchmarking comparison of Premier Multispecialty Group staffing FTE to two output measures—Relative Value Units and Patients—is provided below.

Premier Multispecialty Group
Total Relative Value Units: 66,391
Total Patients: 15,360

Based on this level of analysis, there may be a rightsizing opportunity based on level of outputs as measured by relative value units and patients (Table 6.5). (Careful interpretation is warranted, however, as the MGMA benchmark data include staffing categories that are not incurred by Premier Multispecialty Group.)

TABLE 6.5 Benchmarking Staff Based on Various Outputs

	Premier	MGMA Median
Total Support Staff per 10,000 RVUs	3.77	4.29
Total Support Staff per 10,000 Patients	16.23	20.31

Source: *MGMA Cost Survey: 2001 Report Based on 2000 Data.* Multispecialty Practice, Primary Care Only, Not Owned by Hospital or Integrated Delivery System.

4. Staff FTE per Various Inputs, such as Specialty, Facility Square Footage

Premier Multispecialty Group practices in a 15,360 square foot facility. Due to the size of the facility, different staffing patterns may be warranted to actually staff the physical space. Sharing of staffing resources may be limited based upon facility design and layout and/or staffing may need to be replicated throughout a practice depending upon the space configuration.

Based on this important input, there is a potential opportunity for rightsizing staff (Table 6.6); however, careful interpretation is again warranted since Premier Multispecialty Group does not report all job categories included in the benchmark source.

TABLE 6.6 Benchmarking Staff Based on Various Inputs

	Premier	MGMA Median
Total Support Staff per 10,000 Square Feet	16.67	29.00

Source: *MGMA Cost Survey: 2001 Report Based on 2000 Data,* Multispecialty Practice, Primary Care Only, Not Owned by a Hospital or Integrated Delivery System.

5. Staff FTE Cost per Physician FTE

To compute this measure, FTE staff cost per FTE physician, staff compensation for each staffing category is determined and then calculated on a per FTE physician basis. This is then compared to benchmark levels to determine if there is opportunity related to skill mix, wage rates or staffing levels based on the expenditures associated with staffing Premier Multispecialty Group.

This level of analysis reveals that the expenditure levels by Premier Multispecialty Group on a per FTE physician basis for administrative and business office staff and for front office

TABLE 6.7 ■ Benchmarking Staff Cost by Staffing Category

Staff Category	Premier Total Cost	Premier Cost Per FTE Physician	MGMA Median
Administrative & Business Staff	$155,000	$22,142	$32,035
Front Office Staff	$115,000	$16,429	$33,052
Clinical Staff	$299,500	$42,785	$43,695
Ancillary Service Staff	$85,000	$12,143	$13,839
TOTAL	$850,850	$121,549	$149,880

Source: Appendix III, Table 4e. Data derived from MGMA *Cost Survey: 2001 Report Based on 2000 Data*, Multispecialty Practices with Primary Care Only, Not Owned by Hospital or Integrated Delivery System.

staff are below median benchmark norms. Expenditure levels for clinical support staff and ancillary service staff, however, are consistent with the median benchmarks.

Table 6.8 proceeds to a more detailed analysis and reflects staffing expenditures at the job classification level.

TABLE 6.8 ■ Benchmarking Staff Cost Based on Staffing Classification Level

Staff Title	Premier Total Cost	Premier Per FTE Physician	MGMA Median
Administrative & Business Staff			
General Administrative	$80,000	$11,428	$13,708
Business Office	$75,000	$10,714	$17,252
Managed Care	$.00	$.00	$5,458
Information Technology	$.00	$.00	$3,716
Housekeeping/Maintenance/Security	$.00	$.00	$2,978
Front Office & Clerical Staff			
Medical Receptionists	$99,000	$14,143	$20,448
Medical Secretaries/Transcribers	$.00	$.00	$6,195
Medical Records	$16,000	$2,286	$5,000
Other Administrative Support	$.00	$.00	$4,362
Clinical Support Staff			
Registered Nurses	$87,500	$12,500	$13,010
Licensed Practical Nurses	$162,500	$23,214	$10,991
Medical Assistants, Aides	$49,500	$7,071	$13,704
Ancillary Staff			
Clinical Laboratory	$50,000	$7,143	$9,835
Radiology and Imaging	$35,000	$5,000	$6,358
Other Medical Support	$0.00	$0.00	$3,471
Total Employed Staff	***$654,500***	***$93,499***	***$123,979***
Contracted Support Staff	***$0.00***	***$0.00***	***$4,829***
Total Benefits	***$196,350***	***$28,050***	***$25,615***
Total Support Staff	***$850,850***	***$121,549***	***$149,880***

Source: Appendix III, Table 4b. Data derived from MGMA *Cost Survey: 2001 Report Based on 2000 Data*, Multispecialty Practices with Primary Care Only, Not Owned by Hospital or Integrated Delivery System.

At this level of analysis, Premier Multispecialty Group is spending less dollars for staffing on a per FTE physician basis than its benchmark counterparts. It is important to examine this data at the specific job classification level, as Premier does not report certain job categories that are included in the benchmark source. Analysis of staffing cost at the job classification level permits opportunities to identify rightsizing relative to staff support cost based upon skill mix, staffing levels, wage levels and benefit costs.

6. Staff Cost As a Percent of Total Medical Revenue

In this final quantitative benchmark measure, staffing cost as a percent of total medical revenue is computed. As discussed previously, this measure reflects not only the level of staff, but the contribution of staff to overall profitability. Better performing medical groups generally report higher levels of staff and higher cost of staff per FTE physician, but have lower staff cost as a percent of total medical revenue.

Premier Multispecialty Group: Annual Total Medical Revenue: $2,100,000

The contribution of staffing to practice profitability was detailed earlier in this text. Based on staffing expenditure levels as a percent of total medical revenue, there is clear opportunity for Premier Multispecialty Group. While earlier benchmarking reflected clinical support and ancillary services staffing levels consistent with benchmark normative data, the cost of these categories of staff are higher for Premier Multispecialty Group as a percent of total medical revenue. This suggests an opportunity to investigate the staff contribution to the practice's profitability. That is, are these employees doing the right things to support practice efficiency and profitability? The next table examines staff cost as a percent of total medical revenue at the job classification level.

At this level of analysis, it is apparent that Premier Multispecialty Group is spending more dollars on staffing as a percent of total medical revenue than benchmark norms in a number of job classification areas. This suggests opportunities to rightsize staff; however, this finding should not preclude investigation of other areas, such as billing and collection performance, payer mix of the practice, physician coding variability, etc. that may impact the denominator (total medical revenue).

TABLE 6.9 ■ Benchmarking Staff Based on Cost As a Percent of Total Medical Revenue by Staffing Category

Staff Category	Premier Total Cost	Premier Cost as a Percent of Total Medical Revenue	MGMA Median
Administrative & Business Staff	$155,000	7.38%	6.53%
Front Office Staff	$115,000	5.47%	7.42%
Clinical Staff	$299,500	14.27%	8.46%
Ancillary Service Staff	$85,000	4.05%	3.10%
TOTAL	$850,850	40.52%	29.98%

Source: Appendix III, Table 4f. Data derived from MGMA *Cost Survey: 2001 Report Based on 2000 Data*, Multispecialty Practices with Primary Care Only, Not Owned by Hospital or Integrated Delivery System.

TABLE 6.10 ■ Benchmarking Staff Cost As a Percent of Total Medical Revenue Based on Staffing Classification Level

Staff Title	Premier Total Cost	Premier Total Cost as a % of Total Medical Revenue	MGMA Median
Administrative & Business Staff			
General administrative	$80,000	3.81%	2.97%
Business office	$75,000	3.57%	3.53%
Managed care	$0.00	0.00%	1.23%
Information technology	$0.00	0.00%	0.65%
Housekeeping/maintenance/security	$0.00	0.00%	0.52%
Front Office & Clerical Staff			
Medical receptionists	$99,000	4.71%	3.93%
Medical secretaries/transcribers	$0.00	0.00%	1.16%
Medical records	$16,000	0.76%	1.07%
Other administrative support	$0.00	0.00%	0.74%
Clinical Support Staff			
Registered nurses	$87,500	4.17%	2.47%
Licensed practical nurses	$162,500	7.74%	2.90%
Medical assistants, aides	$49,500	2.36%	2.90%
Ancillary Staff			
Clinical laboratory	$50,000	2.38%	1.90%
Radiology and imaging	$35,000	1.67%	1.31%
Other medical support	$0.00	0.00%	0.69%
Total employed staff	**$654,500**	**31.17%**	**25.01%**
Contracted support staff	$0.00	0.00%	0.97%
Total benefits	**$196,350**	**9.35%**	**5.51%**
Total support staff	**$850,850**	**40.52%**	**29.98%**

Source: Appendix III, Table 4. Data derived from MGMA *Cost Survey: 2001 Report Based on 2000 Data*, Multispecialty Practices with Primary Care Only, Not Owned by Hospital or Integrated Delivery System.

As demonstrated by this case study, the first step in the staff rightsizing process—Benchmark the Current State—permits a comparison of the medical practice's current staffing levels, skill mix, and staffing cost with peer groups and with better performing medical practices. Through this analysis, areas of opportunity emerge that receive focused attention during the next steps of the staff rightsizing process.

■ STEP 2: ANALYZE CURRENT PRODUCTIVITY

Step 2 in the rightsizing process involves understanding the current productivity levels of the support staff in the medical practice. In order to determine whether an employee is performing at optimal productivity levels, expected workload ranges for a particular function or task need to be established, with current staff productivity measured and compared against this workload range.

In Step 2, data are collected regarding the current productivity of staff in the performance of a specific work function. The next step is to determine the expected workload range for this function. This involves actual observation of the work tasks required to perform the function, with an estimate as to the time required for each of the work tasks. Expected workload ranges should be established for each critical business process in the practice, so that a gap analysis can be performed between current and expected productivity levels.

FIGURE 6.4 ■ Questions for Rightsizing Step 2

> **Step 2: Analyze Current Productivity**
> 1. What are the staffing utilization levels for critical work processes?
> 2. Is more or less support staff needed to perform these functions if the current work process is not changed?
> 3. What are the expected performance outcomes? Have they been met?

The questions addressed in Step 2 of the rightsizing process are outlined in Figure 6.4.

It is important that this step be carefully applied, as employees in the medical practice are clearly not robots. Medical practice employees are knowledge workers involved in a service industry, not a manufacturing production line. It would be appropriate to consider building non-productive time into the workload ranges, for example, a 20 percent reduction for non-productive time to recognize the interruptions and unplanned events that occur throughout the day in a medical practice environment. In addition, if trade-offs between quantity and quality need to be made, quality clearly needs to have priority emphasis in a medical practice.

The steps in this phase of the rightsizing process include:

1. Determining the function or task to be studied;
2. Collecting data;
3. Identifying expected workload ranges; and
4. Analyzing performance gaps.

The following four examples are provided to illustrate analysis of current productivity in a medical practice.

EXAMPLE 1: STAFF PRODUCTIVITY ANALYSIS—ACCOUNT FOLLOW-UP

Suppose that a medical practice wants to determine whether billing account follow-up coordinators are working at optimal levels. The first step is to collect data regarding current staff productivity for a typical one-week period as follows:

Account Follow-up Coordinator
Day 1:   50 accounts followed in 6 hours
Day 2:   60 accounts followed in 6.5 hours
Day 3:   50 accounts followed in 6 hours
Day 4:   55 accounts followed in 5.5 hours
Day 5:   50 accounts followed in 6 hours
Total 5 Days: 265 accounts followed in 30 hours or an average of 9 per hour

The next step is to determine the expected workload range for this function. This involves actual observation of the work tasks required to perform account follow-up, with an estimate as to the time required for each of the work tasks. In reviewing this task, a practice executive may determine that the expected workload range for account follow-up is 70 to 105 accounts worked per day or 10 to 15 per hour. A comparison of the current productivity level of the staff with the expected productivity level can now be performed. In this example, the current staff utilization based on the expected workload range is 60 to 90 percent.

There could be a variety of factors that impact the ability to perform within the expected range. For example, perhaps the accounts are old and require extensive building of account history prior to follow-up. Questions the practice might ask include:

- Is there an opportunity for improvement?
- Has technology been appropriately leveraged for this function, for example, is there an automated system for account follow-up?
- Is the practice limited to three accounts per telephone call with the insurance carrier or has the practice attempted to develop a relationship with the payer, for example, a scheduled two-hour conference call each week to follow-up on the accounts?
- Can the process be streamlined?

EXAMPLE 2: STAFF PRODUCTIVITY ANALYSIS—PAYMENT POSTING

If the performance workload range that is adopted for payment posting is 500 to 600 payment posting transactions per day, and the payment poster can only seem to post 100 to 125 per day, this represents a staffing utilization of approximately 20 percent. This analysis permits the medical practice executive to then explore why the staff member is unable to perform within the expected workload range. For example, if a staff member posts to 45 separate databases, it would require more time to post payments than a staff member who only posts to one database that has a shared registration. If payment posters are line item posting, it may take a longer time than balance forward posting, and obviously this would impact the workload range. If there have been payment posting inaccuracies in the past, this could also impact the time required to effectively post the payment to the account as the payment poster must reconstruct the account history prior to posting the payment.

EXAMPLE 3: STAFF PRODUCTIVITY ANALYSIS—WORKING THE CREDIT BALANCE REPORT

How many staff does it take to work the credit balance report? Let's assume that a medical practice has 2,500 accounts in credit balance status that need to be worked. If an expected workload range is 10 to 12 minutes to work each account (to review the account, investigate it, obtain a copy of the explanation of benefits, copy the backup, prepare a refund request, etc), it is possible to determine the staffing needed to fully work the report. For example:

2,500 accounts X 10 minutes = 25,000 minutes = 417 hours
2,500 accounts X 12 minutes = 30,000 minutes = 500 hours
Range: 417-500 hours to work the credit balance report

EXAMPLE 4: STAFF PRODUCTIVITY ANALYSIS—PATIENT RECEPTION

Are the receptionists working at optimal levels? The first step is to determine the current staffing productivity levels. Then the practice will want to identify the work tasks required for this function and then estimate the time required for each of the tasks in order to develop the expected performance workload range. For example, an observation of the staff member could reveal that it takes about three minutes to perform registration—two minutes to check-out the patient and two minutes to conduct charge entry per visit. That would mean that the expected workload range for the receptionist is approximately 60 to 80 patients per day, per receptionist. If the medical practice has 12,500 visits a year or 50 visits per day (assuming 250 work days per year) and has two receptionists, each receptionist is handling approximately 25 patients per day. The staffing utilization would be approximately 31 to 42 percent.

Questions that could be generated based on this finding:

- Are there a large number of new patients that may take more time than established patients at check-in?
- Is there more that can be done during the pre-visit process, such as obtaining completed paperwork and updating insurance and demographic information, rather than waiting for the patient to present for appointment?
- Is there a large volume of walk-in patients that would impact the staff member's ability to meet the expected performance range?

Step 2 of the staff rightsizing process permits medical practices to understand the productivity levels of staff in the performance of their current work processes. Opportunities to enhance staff productivity and efficiency can then be explored via the next two steps in the rightsizing process: Step 3—Analyze the Current Practice Model and Step 4—Analyze Process Performance.

STEP 3: ANALYZE THE CURRENT PRACTICE MODEL

As detailed in Chapter 5, the practice model that is embraced by the physicians and leaders of the medical practice has a significant impact on staffing levels, staffing cost, and staffing workload and tasks. The reader is encouraged to review the five sample practice models that were previously outlined in Chapter 5 in order to recognize the impact of the models on staffing and clinical support to physicians.

Many practices have not taken advantage of economies of scale in their group practice configurations. For example, co-locating six physicians in a physical office setting, but continuing to maintain each of the individual physician's practices as an independent, autonomous entity will require a different level of staffing than if the physicians are practicing in a true group practice model.

Questions to be addressed during Step 3 in the rightsizing process include the following:

1. What type of practice model has been embraced? This may require an operations assessment of a representative sampling of the medical group's outpatient sites to identify the practice model(s) that is currently in place.

2. What is the purpose of the current practice model? That is, was the model selected consistent with a particular business plan? If so, has the model achieved the expected performance outcomes? For example, if multiple practice sites were established to provide patient outreach opportunities and to serve as "feeder" systems to the hospital as part of a competitive market share positioning strategy, is the cost/benefit analysis still valid? If this goal has been achieved, would it be beneficial to review the geographic distribution of practice sites via a formal regional model of care delivery?

FIGURE 6.5 ■ Questions for Rightsizing Step 3

> **Step 3: Analyze the Practice Model**
> 1. What type of practice model has been embraced?
> 2. What is the purpose of the current model?
> 3. Is there another practice model that could enhance efficiency and service?
> 4. Is the facility presenting a limitation for efficient practice?
> 5. Is the medical practice taking advantage of economies of scale?
> 6. What duties have been delegated to staff?
> 7. To what extent have functions been shared or distributed?
> 8. Who are the key parties to involve in model discussions?

3. Is there another practice model that could enhance physician productivity and efficiency and meet patient service expectations?
4. Is the facility itself presenting a limitation for efficient practice? For example, a large multispecialty practice occupying three floors of a medical office building may currently be configured to allow for eight separate reception areas and check-in stations, when a different patient flow process might permit economies of scale.
5. Is the medical practice organized to take advantage of economies of scale (or simply supporting individual practices that have been co-located)? For example, are 6 to 8 providers practicing in a suite a full five days each week?
6. What duties have been delegated to the staff? For example, is nursing staff expected to room patients, manage telephone calls, triage patients, handle prescription refills, etc., or are separate staff involved in these duties? Are physicians delegating appropriate work to clinical support staff?
7. To what extent have specific functions and tasks been shared or distributed throughout the practice? For example, is there a central check-in/check-out area or are these functions distributed throughout the practice suites in the building? Do nurses support more than one provider? Is there a systematic process to handle prescription refills and test results reporting?
8. Who are the key parties to involve in discussions of the advantages and disadvantages of alternative practice models?

■ STEP 4: ANALYZE PROCESS PERFORMANCE

The fourth step in the rightsizing process involves analyzing process performance. If a particular work process is highly encumbered in comparison to other practices, requiring multiple process steps and hand-offs, a higher staffing level may be required, simply due to the added complexity of the work process itself. As we indicated earlier, it is the processes that produce the costs, not the staff. If key processes in a medical practice are encumbered, additional employees may be needed in order to perform effectively. Questions asked during Step 4 of the rightsizing process are outlined in Figure 6.6.

FIGURE 6.6 ■ Questions for Rightsizing Step 4

> **Step 4: Analyze Process Performance**
> 1. What is the goal of this particular process?
> 2. What are the boundaries of the process?
> 3. What is the current process?
> 4. What are the process measures?
> 5. Is there a better way to perform this process?

The steps used in analyzing process performance include:

1. Select a key business process;
2. Bound the process—identify where the process starts and where it ends;
3. Flowchart and/or measure the current process;
4. Identify areas of opportunity.

To understand process variability, four examples are offered to assist in adopting the lens of an observer to the medical practice. Adopting the observer lens is often difficult for process owners, those individuals who created the current process that is being examined.

EXAMPLE 1: ANALYZE PROCESS PERFORMANCE—THE PATIENT SCHEDULING PROCESS

The next two figures (Figures 6.7 and 6.8) contain very different flowcharts of a patient scheduling process.

FIGURE 6.7 ■ Patient Scheduling Process A

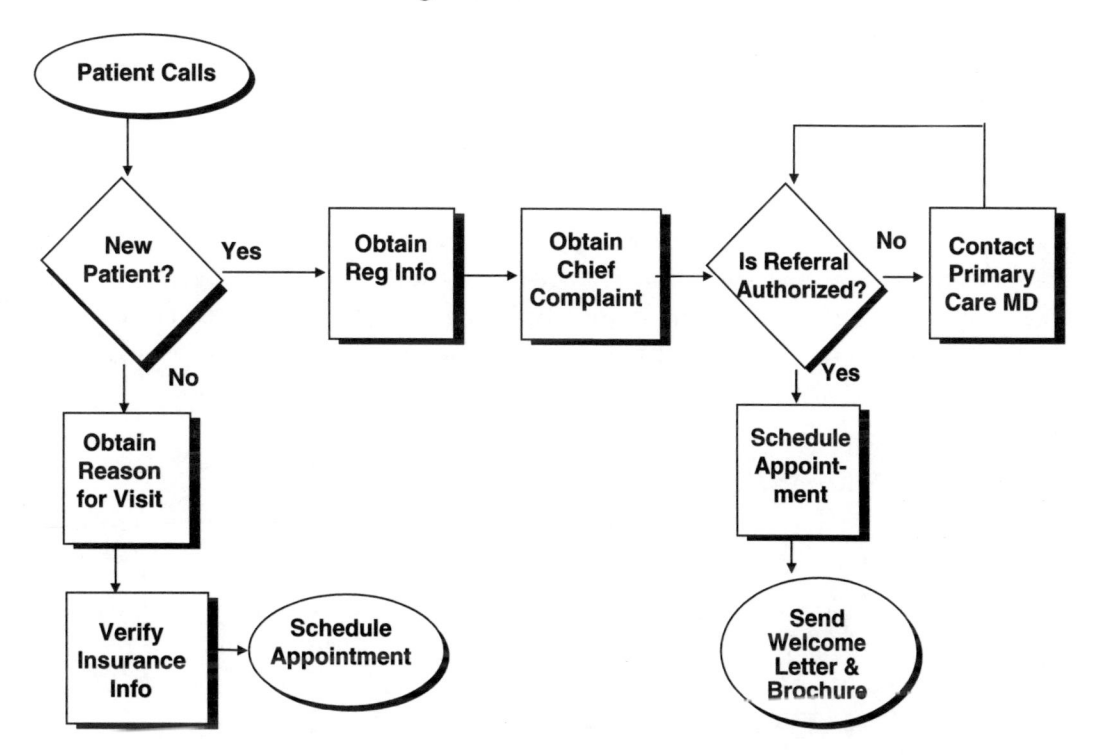

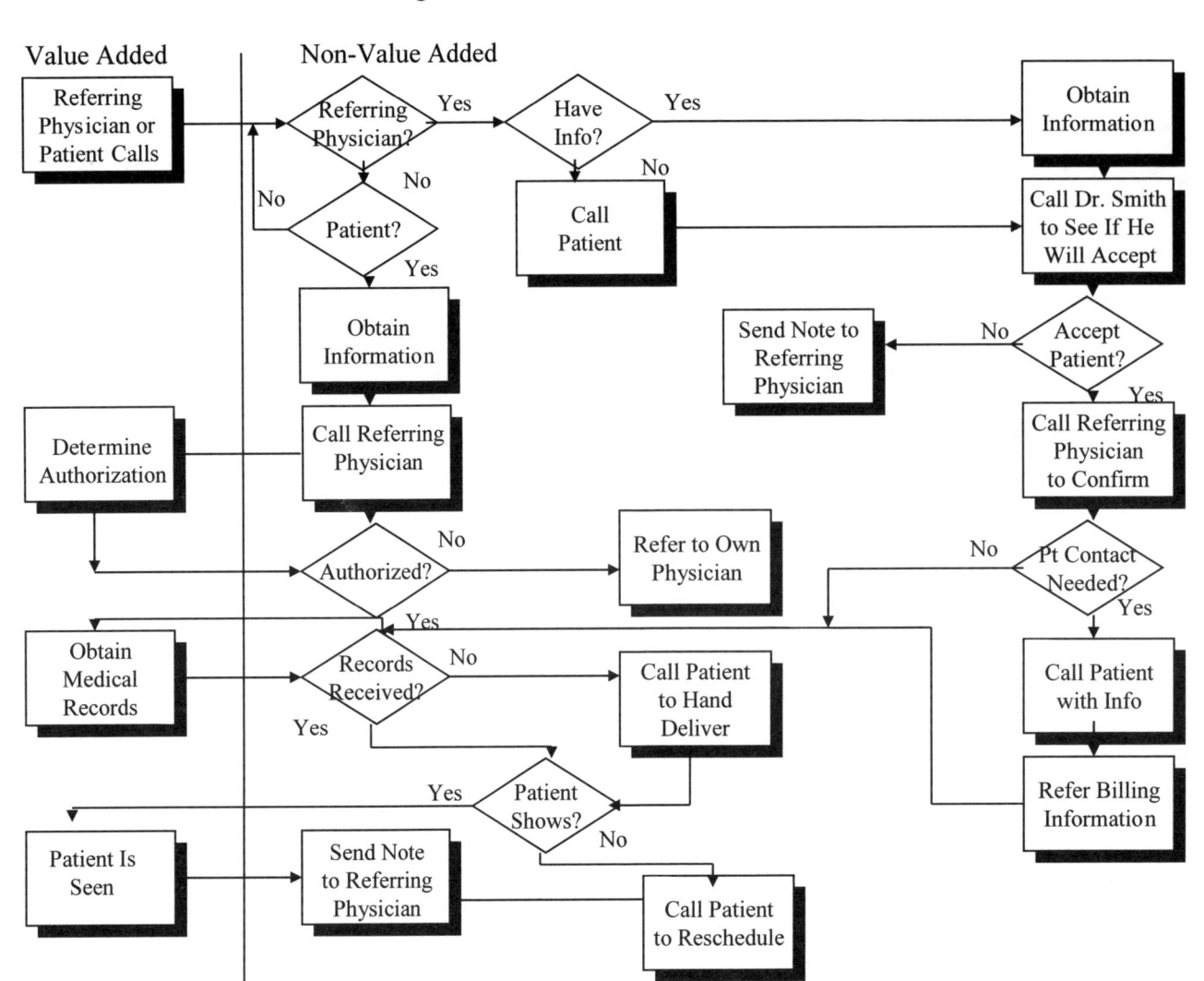

FIGURE 6.8 ■ Patient Scheduling Process B

Observation: It is obvious that Patient Scheduling Process A is streamlined, while Patient Scheduling Process B is highly encumbered. Patient Scheduling Process B contains a number of steps that are non-value added for the patient. These additional steps create complexity in the process and more scheduling staff will be required to perform this process.

Via similar flowcharting and analysis, each of the critical processes in a medical practice can be reviewed and analyzed for areas of opportunity. Questions that should be asked include:

1. What is value-added from the patient's perspective?
2. What is considered non-valued added, and how can that be streamlined and/or eliminated?
3. What are the current process measures? Process measures include process steps, decision-points, hand-offs, and cycle time. Cycle time is the time required for the entire process to be completed from start to finish.
4. Are the process measures within acceptable thresholds/levels?

5. Is there a better way to meet customer needs (both external customers: patients, referring physicians, health plans, and employers and internal customers: physicians, midlevel providers, and support staff) by streamlining or innovating the process?
6. Would a change to the practice model permit opportunities to improve the process, for example, linking tasks, consolidating functions, moving steps up into the pre-visit process, changing the patient flow process, adopting a group practice perspective, centralizing scheduling and referral, etc.

These questions may lead to site visits or networking with colleagues to determine if they have adopted a more innovative or streamlined process for this function.

EXAMPLE 2: ANALYZE PROCESS PERFORMANCE—CLINICAL SUPPORT

Observation: A pediatric practice employs a full-time registered nurse to administer allergy shots. In addition, each of the 4.00 FTE physicians have a full-time (1.00 FTE) LPN.

Here are some questions that should be asked related to the current staffing pattern and work process in order to understand the current process and determine if there is opportunity to improve the process for the future:

1. Is a registered nurse needed to administer allergy shots?
2. How many allergy shots are administered? What is the patient load each day by time of day?
3. Does each physician work 10 sessions per week? Do they see similar patient volumes? Is patient severity of illness/acuity similar?
4. Are LPN employees performing duties at the level of their licensure?
5. Does each physician need a 1.00 LPN or could a different staffing strategy be a better use of practice resources and still support physician productivity and patient service?

EXAMPLE 3: ANALYZE PROCESS PERFORMANCE—PHYSICIAN INTERRUPTED

Observation: In this particular practice, the physician takes telephone calls on average 10 minutes each hour, or 80 minutes each day. We can actually estimate the cost of this activity by minute.

Physician Salary: $240,000
Physician Benefits: $48,000
Total: $288,000
Cost/Minute: $2.40
(assumes 40 hours/week * 50 weeks/year* 60 minutes/hour) = 120,000)
Cost/Day: $192.00   Cost/Week: $960.00   Cost/Year: $48,000

Questions that should be addressed when analyzing this process:

1. What type of inbound telephone calls is the physician receiving?
2. Can someone else in the practice respond to the calls, such as nurse triage staff?
3. Does the $48,000 justify a nurse triage position?

It is important to recognize the "opportunity costs" associated with this telephone workload for the physician. The physician could generate significant patient access opportunity and revenue by seeing patients during this 80-minute period if the calls could be reduced and/or eliminated. If the physician sees patients every 10 minutes, eight additional patients could be seen. If the physician schedules patients every 15 minutes, an additional five patients per day could be seen. In addition, nurse triage may reduce unnecessary patient visits and permit the physician to see patients of higher acuity.

EXAMPLE 4: ANALYZE PROCESS PERFORMANCE—TELEPHONE MANAGEMENT

Observation: In this example, the practice employs five telephone operators and each employee works from 8:00 a.m. to 5:00 p.m. each day. The phones are transferred to an answering service during the lunch hour.

In order to analyze the telephone management process for this practice, the following types of questions should be addressed:

1. What is the inbound telephone volume by time of day and day of week?

2. What type of inbound telephone calls are received (schedule appointment, talk to nurse, prescription refill, etc.)?

3. Can inbound telephone demand be minimized? That is, are there other ways that patients' needs can be addressed rather than incur a random or episodic call volume throughout the day. For example, many practices ask patients to contact their pharmacy directly for prescription refills, with the pharmacy interacting with the practice via fax. Medical records personnel then pick up the fax requests at systematic intervals throughout the day, for example, at 10:00 a.m., 12:00 noon, 2:00 p.m. and 4:00 p.m., pull the medical records, and deliver the chart and pharmacy faxes to the nursing area. This minimizes process steps and process hand-offs, and permits a focused attention to prescription refill requests. Other practices have an automated line for messages related to prescriptions, with staff transcribing the messages at systematic times throughout the day.

4. Why are the telephones transferred during lunch? Patients may want to contact physician offices during the noon hour when they have work breaks of their own. Transferring the calls essentially represents delaying work rather than performing work in real time.

5. Is a constant staffing pattern throughout the week warranted based on the data? That is, suppose that this practice has the typical pattern of a high volume of telephone calls on Monday morning and again on Friday late afternoon. If the practice has been staffing at a constant level, such as 8:00 a.m.–5:00 p.m. Monday through Friday, perhaps there is opportunity for more flexible staffing deployment consistent with the variation in workload.

Beyond the above analysis of process performance, it is important for medical practices to articulate expectations for process performance, so that a current process can be regularly monitored and measured to identify deviation from the expected levels. For example, if a medical practice expects patients to wait a maximum of 20 minutes in the reception area, what is the range and average waiting times actually occurring each day? As another example, if a medical practice expects the medical record to be available 98 percent of the time the patient is seen, and the current availability is 75 percent, this needs to be investigated.

In the latter example, if a staff reduction has recently occurred and the medical record availability dropped from 98 percent to 75 percent, it is important to identify the associated costs of this change to staffing the medical records department. For example, how much of the physician's time is required to rebuild the patient history when the physician does not have the medical record? Is patient care being compromised by not having the chart readily available for the visit? When the chart is available, are all records and reports typically filed in the chart so that the physician does not have to exit the exam room during the patient visit and thereby decrease his/her efficiency?

STEP 5: TAKE ACTION

The last step in the rightsizing process is to take action. Examples of action steps include:

1. Share Data

Data should be shared with physicians and staff at frequent intervals. For example, compare the medical practice's current staffing levels and skill mix with the benchmarking data, demonstrate variation in individual physician productivity and group profitability due to the current staffing plan, or support a new staffing strategy by projecting the associated productivity and profitability gains for the practice. Open communication and access to data are important to (1) educating physicians and staff about business of medicine issues and (2) creating a learning organization that anticipates the need for change in response to the dynamic health care environment.

2. Model Staffing Plans

Model different staffing plans and identify the pros and cons of each plan for the physicians. There is typically more than one staffing plan that will accomplish the practice's goals and objectives. By modeling different staffing plans, the medical practice can see the impact of its current practice model on staffing and explore alternatives that may enhance productivity, efficiency, and performance.

3. Measure the Impact of Staffing Changes

Before and after measures are needed in order to demonstrate that changes to staffing levels, skill mix, work processes or practice models had their intended effect. Types of measures

FIGURE 6.9 ■ Step 5: Take Action

Step 5: Take Action
1. Share Data
2. Model Staffing Plans
3. Measure the Impact of Staffing Changes
4. Adopt "Organized Abandonment" of the Status Quo

include patient satisfaction scores, physician productivity, staffing costs as a percent of total medical revenue, and revenue after operating costs.

4. Adopt "Organized Abandonment" of the Status Quo

Peter Drucker has well-documented the difficulties in changing processes that have been entrenched in the organization.[12] By practicing what Drucker terms "systematic abandonment of the status quo," opportunities to explore better performing medical groups, question current practices and processes, review current forms, and other activities take place in an atmosphere where change is expected.

For example, a medical practice can select one work process to review each quarter, with the benchmarking and rightsizing steps used to determine whether a) the process needs to continue, b) whether there is a better way to perform the process, and c) whether the process is rightsized. By continuing this process each quarter, a culture is created that involves questioning the status quo systematically and at regular intervals. Change simply becomes "the way we do things around here" rather than be viewed as a major disruptive event in the practice.

---

[12]Drucker, PF. The Theory of the Business. Harvard Business Review, Sept.-Oct. 1994; 72(5):95-104

A Closer Look at Staffing Categories and Staffing Models

CHAPTER 7

As staff rightsizing takes place in the medical practice, specific staffing categories need to be investigated to determine if a more appropriate staffing model or staffing work assignment will enhance practice efficiency, productivity, profitability or performance. In the following chapter, key considerations for staffing the major job categories in medical practices are outlined. In addition, outsourcing of work functions and staffing for seasonality involving fluctuations in patient demand are addressed.

In many staffing categories, it is appropriate to assume a "job function approach" to staffing consistent with Step 2 of the rightsizing process that involves analyzing current staff productivity. This requires that the medical practice (1) identify the performance workload ranges specific to its technology and current work processes and (2) identify the appropriate number of staff and skill level of staff required for the particular job function (or alternatively, change the current process to streamline it or remove non-value added steps and then re-assess staffing needs). This job function approach to staffing is demonstrated in a number of the staffing categories discussed in this chapter.

■ GENERAL ADMINISTRATIVE STAFF

Key considerations when addressing rightsizing of general administrative staff include the following:

1. Impacts to Physician Efficiency

Medical practices that are "wrongsized" in the area of general administrative support and have too few administrative staff often experience lower levels of physician efficiency and productivity. This is likely due to the fact that physicians in these types of practices are more actively involved in administrative, non-clinical tasks than their physician counterparts. It may be that by providing enhanced administrative and managerial expertise, physicians can benefit not only from this added attention and expertise to "business of medicine" issues, but also from additional time devoted to clinical practice.

2. The General Administrative Staff Category Extends Beyond Practice Managers and Practice Administrators

Some medical practices that have a central business office have failed to include these staff numbers and costs when benchmarking staffing to the MGMA benchmarking sources. The general administrative staff category as defined by MGMA includes administrators, assistant administrators, chief financial officers, medical directors, directors of nursing, site managers, human resources staff, marketing staff and purchasing department staff. Thus, it is important to include all general administrative staff when benchmarking staffing and performing staff rightsizing.

3. Business Risk

Medical practices that do not have sophisticated medical practice executives may be placing themselves at an unnecessary business risk. The dramatic changes in the health care environment have necessitated a new way of approaching the practice of medicine. Tolerance bands have been narrowed by federal and state agencies, and there is heightened scrutiny regarding billing and collection, contract management, patient confidentiality, records security and other areas related to the delivery of health care services. Beyond the business risk associated with federal and state legal and regulatory requirements, many practices have not been able to maintain current knowledge with regard to labor and personnel issues, medical records management and retention, and other business and administrative areas, thereby enhancing risk to the medical practice.

BILLING OFFICE STAFF

Billing responsibilities have transitioned from a back office function to involve all providers and staff in the medical practice. The "end-to-end" billing process begins at the time the contract is signed with the health plan and ends at the time payment is received, posted, and deposited from an adjudicated claim. Some key considerations when staffing the billing office follow:

1. Assume a Job Function Approach to Staffing

When staffing the billing office, take a job function approach to determine the number of staff required for each major functional area of the billing and collection process. This will require the medical practice to identify performance workload ranges specific to its technology and work processes and then to identify the appropriate number of staff and skill level of staff required for the particular function to be performed.

As an example, suppose the medical practice executive seeks to rightsize the insurance or account follow-up staff. Adopting a job function approach to staffing requires that the staff member be observed performing this function using the medical practice's own technology, work processes, and status of its accounts receivable. A typical time to fully work an account may be found to be four to six minutes per account in order to meet the practice's expectations with regard to performance quality. At this rate, the account follow-up representative is able to work 10 to 15 accounts per hour or 70 to 105 accounts per day. If the medical practice has 5,000 insurance accounts in the over 90 day aging category to be worked each month, then this particular work function would need to be staffed by approximately 2.75

FTE staff. The work conducted by these staff needs to be monitored and measured to determine if the workload range continues to be appropriate and the expectations for work quality are being met.

Note that the performance workload range was first identified by observing a staff member in the actual performance of this work function. Changes that impact this function will also impact the expected workload range. Examples of these changes include:

1. a new process for account follow-up activity (for example, some practices have developed relationships with health plans that permit scheduled conference calls each week);

2. the ability to leverage technology (such as on-line follow-up efforts or improved practice management system);

3. a reduction in account aging (for example, due to increased collections at the time-of-service or "clean-up" of old accounts receivable); and

4. new staff training and orientation (staff newly assigned to this function would not be expected to perform at optimal levels for a six month period).

Taking a job function approach to staffing the billing office involving both quantitative and qualitative data can be applied to the major billing functions including coding, charge entry, claims and statement generation, payment posting, refund processing, insurance account follow-up and patient account follow-up.

2. CONSIDER THE ENTIRE "END-TO-END" BILLING PROCESS WHEN RIGHTSIZING STAFF

Many medical practices continue to consider only the "back-end" billing process when rightsizing staff in the billing or business office. Back-end billing typically includes all of the billing and collection steps that follow charge entry. It is important to recognize that "front-end" billing functions are part of the billing process. Front-end billing typically includes obtaining patient demographic and insurance information, service capture, coding, time-of-service collections activity and charge entry functions. Consideration of the entire billing process is required to rightsize staff. Medical practices that have been able to provide "clean" front-end billing processes typically are able to reduce their staffing levels devoted to insurance and patient account follow-up activities.

3. DELEGATE SPECIFIC, MEASURABLE TASKS TO EMPLOYEES

Medical practices that have successful billing and collection operations delegate specific, well-defined and measurable tasks to billing office staff, as opposed to a staffing model where there is a high level of multi-tasking and general staff assignments. Specific performance expectations and outcomes are articulated and data are shared with the employees so they can self-manage (with appropriate oversight) as knowledge workers. For example, the patient inquiry process can be assigned to specific individuals who are held accountable for (1) responding to billing inquiries by patients within an acceptable timeframe (typically within 48 hours), (2) identifying opportunities to improve patient service and understandability of patient statements, and other related areas.

As another example, better performing medical practices assign account follow-up activity by payer at higher levels than their counterparts (58.90 percent of better performing medical groups utilized a payer delegation of account follow-up activity in the MGMA

Performance and Practices of Successful Medical Groups: 2001 Report Based on 2000 Data). This develops knowledge experts in payer-specific strategies, permits the medical practice to develop relationships with the health plan, and enables staff members to be held accountable for performance.

FRONT OFFICE STAFF

As noted above, front office staff should be considered when rightsizing staff for the billing process. Beyond capturing and verifying patient demographic and insurance information, collecting co-payments, collecting and receiving charge tickets, obtaining signature waivers and performing charge entry, the front office staff is also expected to welcome the patient to the practice.

1. Assume a Job Function Approach to Staffing

A job function approach to staffing can also be conducted for front office staff. For example, observing the staff member perform his/her job may reveal that it takes about three minutes to perform registration (including verifying insurance and demographic information, copying the insurance card, obtaining patient signatures, collecting and receipting co-payments and patient balances), two minutes to check-out the patient, and two minutes to perform charge entry. That would mean that the expected workload range for the receptionist is approximately 60 to 80 patients per day. If the practice typically averages 250 patient visits on Mondays and 175 patient visits per day Tuesday-Friday, then 3.50 staff FTE are required for this function on Mondays and only 2.50 FTE staff on each of the other weekdays.

2. Attend to Pre-Visit Functions

Due to the changes in health plan reimbursement, most medical practices are involved in detailed referral processes or preauthorization processes. Consequently, the data obtained from the patient are vital to ensuring a "clean claim" as well as ensuring that the appropriate approval processes have taken place prior to the provision of care. Pre-visit functions are now formally being built into the front office staffing strategies of many practices. Pre-visit activities include insurance verification, coverage or pre-authorization for services verification, verification of co-payment levels and patient balances, and demographic or insurance updates that are performed prior to the patient visit. The staffing model used for this function may involve a separate unit, be delegated to the telephone patient schedulers or be handled by reception staff prior to the patient visit depending upon the specialty of the practice, patient volume and practice model that has been adopted.

3. Separate Telephone Management from Reception Functions

Due to heightened knowledge required to perform reception functions and the importance of ensuring data and billing accuracy and patient confidentiality, most medical practices have already or are working to segregate telephone management functions from the front office reception staff. The telephone management functions have also expanded due to pre-visit functions involving insurance verification and due to sophisticated patient scheduling techniques. Thus, strong consideration should be given to a staffing model that segregates telephones from the in-person patient check-in and patient check-out functions.

4. Actively Manage Telephone Demand

Many practices have incorporated an automated attendant feature, eliminating the need for a switchboard operator. The automated attendant can permit a staffing model that supports a systematic approach to handling inbound telephone activity. For example, a prescription refill line can be designated for patients, with calls taken off the line at specific intervals throughout the day, rather than handled episodically. Many practices have been able to optimize the use of pharmaceutical fax or other electronic options, with patients contacting the pharmacy, and the pharmacy contacting the medical practice. The fax machine in the medical practice can be placed in the medical records department with the medical records pulled at regular, systematic intervals and delivered to the nurse with the fax request, minimizing the re-work and hand-offs involved in the prescription refill process.

The reasons for patient inbound telephone calls should be regularly tracked and monitored by reason of call, day of week, and time of day to determine appropriate staffing levels and to actively work to identify the root cause of the patient's need. For example, some patients have been instructed to contact the medical practice if they have not heard the results of their laboratory test in two days when the test itself may take longer to perform. Understanding the reason for the inbound telephone calls will permit proactive steps to be taken to anticipate patient concerns and minimize rework in the practice.

These types of data are also used to take a job function approach to staffing the telephone management process. For example, an observation of telephone operators in the practice may reveal that it takes approximately two minutes for message-taking and approximately three minutes to schedule a patient appointment (with partial registration). Based on the volume and reason for inbound telephone calls, the appropriate staffing levels based on workload can be computed (note that changes to the process, such as electronic chart ordering, electronic message-taking and/or enhanced scheduling software may alter the workload range for the future).

5. Consider Eliminating the Patient Check-out Station

Many practices that collect co-payments at the time of patient arrival have been able to eliminate the patient check-out function altogether. Return patient appointments are made by the clinical support staff, who also give patients written instructions regarding scheduling of tests, procedures, and specialty referrals.

MEDICAL RECORDS STAFF

Staffing for a central medical records unit is based upon work levels. The following areas need to be addressed when rightsizing medical records staff.

1. Assign Staff Based on Work Function

Staff should be assigned based upon work function, not on a per physician or per clinic basis. This permits appropriate monitoring of performance and equitable distribution of workload levels among staff.

Typical work functions in the medical records department include:

1. Filing
2. Chart retrieval, check-out, and re-filing
3. Courier services
4. Records release functions

Expectations for turnaround times for each of these functions should be established, with appropriate monitoring of this activity. One of the primary complaints aired by physicians is the unavailability of patient records and test results. Medical records filing should be given a high priority, with additional resources devoted to filing when it is backlogged beyond acceptable norms.

2. REVIEW COURIER ROLE

Some medical practices ask medical records staff to continually retrieve and deliver charts throughout the day, with charts typically delivered within 10 to 15 minutes for all chart requests. Other practices have recognized that while a STAT request for a medical record may occasionally be needed, a more systematic approach toward chart retrieval and delivery will provide an opportunity for staff to focus on work responsibilities with less interruption to process performance. In these practices, medical records are retrieved and couriered to the practice area(s) on a systematic basis, such as four or five times throughout the day, rather than on a continuous basis.

3. BUILD IN RECORDS PREVIEW FUNCTIONS

Medical records should be previewed prior to the patient visit. This can include multiple levels of review as follows:

1. When charts are pulled for the scheduled patient appointments, the medical records staff should ensure that all material in the record is filed, and that there is no loose paperwork.
2. When charts are provided in the practice site, clinical support staff should review the chart prior to patient presentation to ensure that all test results and records are on the chart. Based upon practice type and volume, some practices have incorporated a formal "chart preview" unit in the medical records area involving clinical support staff who perform this function.
3. Chart preview for account balance, co-payment level, and other business forms should also be conducted prior to the patient visit. Better performing medical practices typically perform this type of chart checking via the practice management software system rather than use the medical record as the source document for this review.

■ CLINICAL SUPPORT STAFF

A question that is frequently posed is "What duties should the nurse perform?" The answer depends upon the practice model that has been embraced. Recognizing that staffing is a measure of work, it is important to identify the skill needs of staff involved in various clinical support functions with the goals of (1) "matching" the staff to the required work function and (2) ensuring expected levels of productivity.

If the medical practice has a one-to-one assignment between the LPN and the physician, the LPN typically would be expected to perform the following types of responsibilities:

- Respond to patient telephone inquiries;
- Process prescription refills;
- Screen laboratory results;
- Mail normal laboratory results to patients;
- Perform clinical pre-visit functions, for example, chart preparation, visit preparation, procedure preparation;
- Room patients for the patient visit;
- Track patient registries and patient logs;
- Process patient referrals;
- Provide patient education; and
- Perform nursing duties such as administering injections, immunizations and wound care.

However, if the medical practice, has (1) a central treatment center which performs injections, immunizations, wound care, and procedures, and (2) dedicated nurse triage staff that are involved in responding to patient telephone inquiries, the duties of the LPN assigned to the physician for patient visit support will need to be redefined. In the latter medical practice, a one-to-one assignment of the LPN to the physician may not be appropriate since the nurse is performing a significantly limited scope of services. In this practice, the clinical support staff is primarily focused on the patient visit process and could conceivably be assigned to two providers (up to six exam rooms).

A key to staffing for clinical support is to identify the practice model and to staff it appropriately, consistent with the workload and needs of physicians and patients. Physician productivity, type of services performed, patient acuity, etc. need to be taken into account. If the practice elects to have centralized nursing functions (for example, telephone nurse triage unit or central treatment area staffed by nurses), then a new role definition and job boundary is required for nurses who assist in the patient visit process to ensure they are performing at acceptable productivity levels.

ANCILLARY STAFF

Practices that have on-site ancillary services—laboratory and radiology—will reflect dissimilar staffing levels when compared to practices that utilize hospital or other resources for these functions. Similar to other staffing categories, the workload levels of staff should be evaluated to determine whether or not the staff is "rightsized" as part of the five-step rightsizing process, however, a financial analysis or return-on-investment associated with these services is also recommended. While patient convenience is an obvious issue, the cost associated with idle ancillary equipment and staff warrants this type of investigation. Many practices began providing radiological services on-site to enhance patient convenience; however, the data simply may not support a cost-effective enterprise and other options to provide these services should be explored.

Key issues to be explored when analyzing ancillary staff levels include:

1. Reception Functions

Are the reception functions for radiology and laboratory services provided at the radiology/laboratory unit or centrally within the medical practice? Some practices that have elected to distribute this function do not have the patient levels to support an entirely separate reception function for these services in the radiology or laboratory department.

2. Duplicate Functions

Are services duplicated in the facility that would be more appropriately consolidated? Some practices provide a separate nursing station for standing orders—for example, involving blood draw—yet also staff a clinical laboratory on-site. As another example, it may be possible to consolidate injections and immunizations, rather than having each nurse responsible for this administration. Note in the latter example, with a focused service approach for these activities, a different skill mix of clinical support for patient visits and/or a different expectation regarding levels of clinical productivity may be warranted.

3. Hours of Availability of Ancillary Services

With many practices electing to expand patient access hours, a return-on-investment analysis is needed to determine whether radiology and clinical laboratory also need to be available during the expanded hours. A number of medical practices have staffed for full ancillary service availability, only to realize that patient volume does not support this level of service and other options may be available for the patient.

4. Integrating Ancillary Services and Service Delivery Models

With on-site laboratories, many practices ask patients to first report to the laboratory 15 minutes prior to their appointment for laboratory work and then report to the practice site for appointment pursuant to established clinical protocols. The laboratory results are transmitted to the physician via fax, printer, or other electronic means within 10 to 15 minutes, to inform the physician during the patient's visit and to electronically link the laboratory test to the practice management software system. This follows an "episode of care" delivery approach to laboratory testing that may lead to enhanced patient flow and practice efficiency (note: this model needs to be consistent with patient care appropriateness and health plan billing requirements). This attempt to integrate ancillary services during the patient visit in an episode of care model is quite different from the historical process typically followed. Process flowcharts for this episode of care process & for the historical process are provided below.

It should be noted that the historical flowchart below represents a streamlined process for ancillary testing and reporting, as many practices incur a number of additional steps in the process, such as the patient calling the practice to request the results before they are available, "telephone tag" to reach the patient, the nurse contacting the laboratory to request test results, multiple attempts to locate the patient's medical records, and other rework steps in the process.

FIGURE 7.1 ■ Two Flowcharts of Ancillary Service

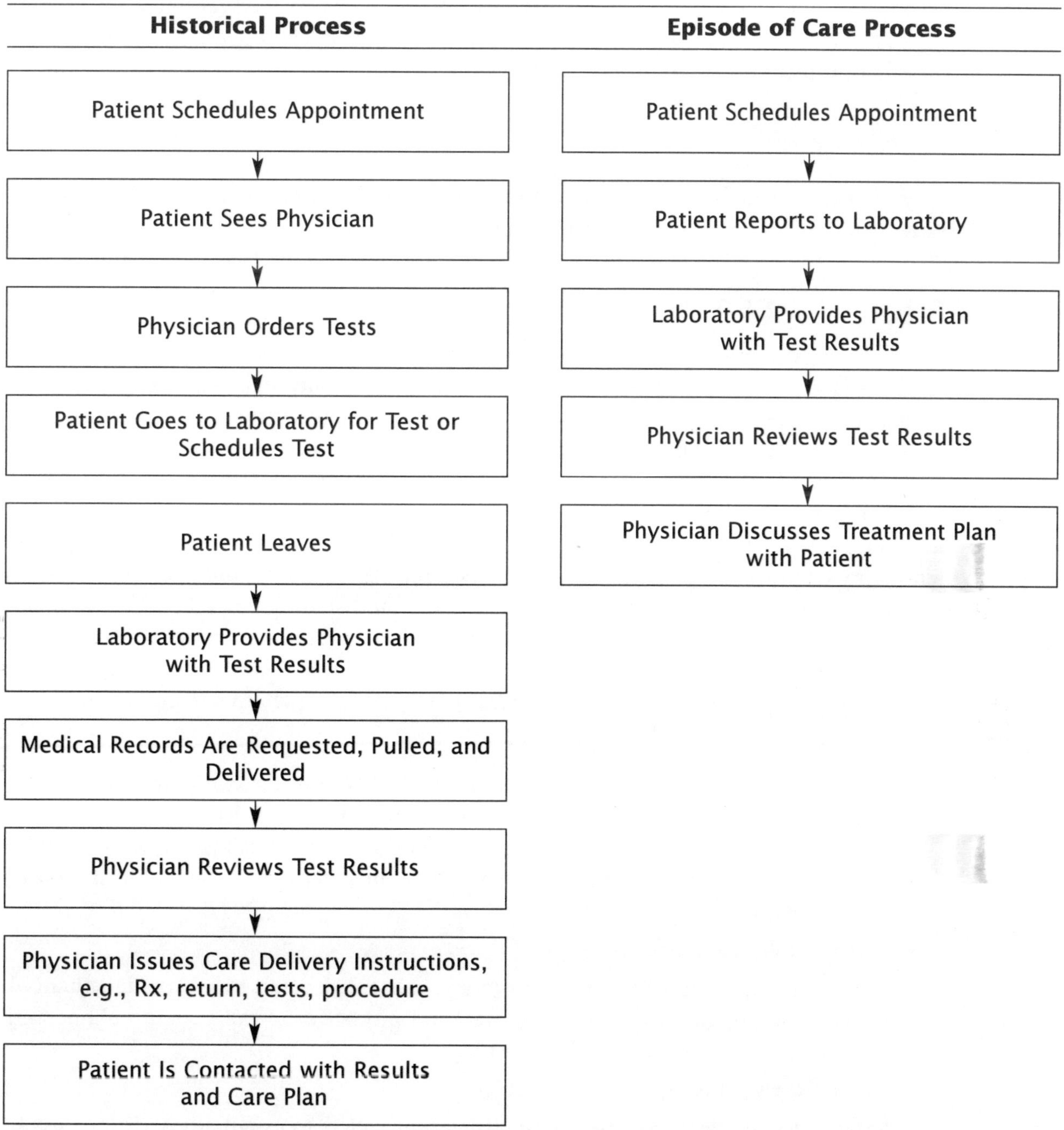

Historical Process

Patient Schedules Appointment
↓
Patient Sees Physician
↓
Physician Orders Tests
↓
Patient Goes to Laboratory for Test or Schedules Test
↓
Patient Leaves
↓
Laboratory Provides Physician with Test Results
↓
Medical Records Are Requested, Pulled, and Delivered
↓
Physician Reviews Test Results
↓
Physician Issues Care Delivery Instructions, e.g., Rx, return, tests, procedure
↓
Patient Is Contacted with Results and Care Plan

Episode of Care Process

Patient Schedules Appointment
↓
Patient Reports to Laboratory
↓
Laboratory Provides Physician with Test Results
↓
Physician Reviews Test Results
↓
Physician Discusses Treatment Plan with Patient

■ OUTSOURCING JOB FUNCTIONS

Outsourcing arrangements contribute to variable staffing levels between medical practices. For example, a medical practice that performs medical transcription and billing functions in-house may have an overall higher staffing level on a per FTE physician or per FTE provider basis than another practice that may outsource these functions. A medical practice that outsources these functions will incur this expense in its general operating cost category, rather than in its staffing cost category.

Job functions that may be outsourced in the practice include business functions such as accounting and legal support, medical records functions such as medical transcription and records storage (electronic and/or physical storage), and technical support functions such as information technology, technologists and other technical support services. Billing functions may also be performed by an in-house billing office or an external vendor.

Better performing medical practices typically do not outsource areas they consider critical to their core competencies. For example, some better performing practices report that they tend to limit outsourcing of billing functions to only a few functions such as patient statement mailing or patient collections support.

STAFFING FOR SEASONALITY

Many practices have more full-time staff than the rightsizing process would suggest, due to the need to respond to high patient demand during seasonality changes, such as flu season or practices located in winter or summer resort destinations. In addition, some practices have added full-time "float" staff to their practice in case they are needed to cover vacation, sick leave, or family leave. These represent high cost staffing models for a medical practice.

There are a number of alternatives to the above staffing plans that can be explored, including part-time "on call" staff, part-time staff with variable hour arrangements, internal temporary employment pools or regional work pools, flexible scheduling and cross coverage arrangements that will reduce staff FTE volumes and staffing costs. In addition, some practices have adopted a different practice model during flu season or at projected high patient demand.

Examples of practice models to respond to fluctuations in patient demand include:

- "AM Fast Track" Clinic

  One of the seasonal practice models is to offer "AM fast track" clinics involving walk-in for sick patients from 7:00 a.m. to 9:00 a.m. with no scheduled appointments during that time. Patients know they can be seen during this established walk-in clinic, thus minimizing both patient telephone calls to the practice and the physician on-call patient volume.

- Enhanced Weekend Access

  Another model to respond to fluctuations in patient demand is to provide enhanced weekend access, thereby minimizing weekend physician on-call patient volume and high patient volumes on Monday mornings.

- Expanded Use of Nonphysician Providers

  Some practices have identified nonphysician providers to essentially staff the "work-in" patients during high peak demands. This permits the physicians to maximally schedule their calendars with patients of higher acuity.

FIGURE 7.2 ■ Staffing for Seasonality

- "AM fast track" clinic
- Enhanced weekend access
- Expanded use of nonphysician providers
- Walk-in facility

- Walk-in Facility

    A final example of a different practice model during fluctuations in patient demand is to devote additional resources to a current walk-in facility or to establish a walk-in facility during the high peak demand in order to enhance patient access.

These types of practice model variations during a seasonal fluctuation in patient demand tend to provide a more systematic approach to handling fluctuating patient volumes, rather than having each physician and his/her associated staff work harder and faster for prolonged periods of time.

Conclusions and Future Implications

"It's really about management, not measurement."[13]

STAFF RETENTION GOES BEYOND RIGHTSIZING

Retaining the best and brightest employees in the medical practice goes well beyond simply "rightsizing." Recruiting talented individuals to the medical practice who can work effectively as a care team is vital to ensuring appropriate staffing for the medical practice. A combination of base salary and tangible and intangible rewards is equally important in retaining highly qualified staff in the medical practice.

However, it should also be noted that the results of many human resources surveys reveal that salary alone is not the primary motivating factor for most employees when it comes to employee retention. A recent study of employee turnover found that money placed fifth on the list of importance for employees. Four values that placed at higher levels of importance were (1) the ability to balance work and outside life, (2) the meaningfulness of work, (3) trust among employees, and (4) the employee's relationships with his/her supervisor/manager.[14] Of each of these values, it would seem that the purpose of medical practices—the meaningfulness of the work in meeting health care needs of communities—should certainly give medical practices some advantage over competing industries for skilled and talented staff. Recognizing and rewarding employees for their contribution to the medical practice goes well beyond rightsizing and must be approached in the same systematic fashion as the rightsizing methodology described in this book.

---

[13]Kaplan RS. Norton DP. The Balanced Scorecard. Boston: Harvard Business School Press; 1996.

[14]Thompson RW. When Bright Lights Beckon, Keeping Top Employees Requires Many Tools. [Internet] PeopleWise. Available from http://www.lexisnexis.com/peoplewise/workforce/know/keeping.shtml.

RIGHTSIZING IS CRITICAL FOR PRODUCTIVITY, PROFITABILITY, AND PERFORMANCE

As we have demonstrated, rightsizing staff in the medical practice is critical for practice productivity, profitability and performance. It is also critical for physician and employee recruitment and retention. As we have demonstrated, a physician's ability to practice efficiently and optimally is impacted by staffing levels, skill mix, practice models, and other important areas involved in the rightsizing process. In addition, not only is employee morale affected by wrongsizing the practice, but problem staffing also impacts patients' perception of service and can enhance business risk. The staff rightsizing process should be approached with careful diligence and it should be conducted following a systematic framework. The benchmarking and productivity analyses should generate positive inquiry into "why" a particular practice might be at variance with benchmarking norms and "how" the practice can learn from its counterparts in order to enhance productivity, profitability and performance.

What Is Our Goal?

The right number of staff, in the right place, with the right skills, at the right cost, with the right behavior, with the right rewards, with the right outcome—no more, no less.

APPENDIXES

Appendix I
Frequently Asked Questions

Answers to frequently asked questions regarding the staff rightsizing process are provided in this Appendix.

1. *What is the definition of a 1.00 FTE physician?*

For purposes of the benchmarking data, what constitutes a 1.00 FTE physician is essentially defined by the practice. That is, if a physician works 35 hours per week in the practice, and this is considered "full-time," then that physician is considered a 1.00 FTE physician. Another practice might expect a 45 hour work week of physicians, and for that practice, the "full time" physician is one who works the full 45 hours each week. This is practice specific. In general, the data in the MGMA *Physician Compensation and Production Survey* treat all physicians equally, if their FTE level ranges from .80 FTE to 1.00 FTE.

2. *Should benchmarking be approached based on patient visits?*

Staffing the medical practice based on patient visits is a good benchmarking approach, but you really want to look at only certain types of staffing in the practice for that comparison. In addition, if benchmarking is based on patient visits alone, it is important to examine critical patient flow and business processes that you actually have in place for your patient visits. If you have encumbered processes, for example, you might be staffing at higher levels than necessary or at higher levels in comparison to peer practices that have successfully streamlined processes, eliminating waste and minimizing non-value added process steps. Staff per visit is an excellent internal metric, something that you can measure internally over time. However, one thing you want to look at is what type of staff you are measuring, because only some of the employees in the practice are really involved in the patient visit. The throughput staff—the receptionist, registered nurses, licensed practical nurses and medical assistants—would make a very good analysis of staffing per patient visit. But other staff, such as business office staff, the executive staff and the administrators in the practice are all relatively fixed until there are major changes in the number of visits.

3. *How can a practice administrator encourage physicians that additional staff will increase profitability and productivity when physicians are typically focused on reducing staff costs?*

The first question to ask the physicians is "What is the goal?" If, in fact, they do want to increase productivity, then perhaps higher levels of staffing may be needed to help them do that. Perhaps some of the physicians may want to leverage their own physician resources via nonphysician providers. If so, the practice will have higher clinical staffing, higher front office staff and higher overhead, but perhaps the net income is going to look terrific. The financial goal of the practice should be to maximize the revenue after operating cost. The medical practice executive will need to model staffing and productivity to help the physicians understand that the increase in compensation and benefit costs will be more than made up by the increased revenue associated with enhanced productivity. This is an important time to look at internal benchmarking where you can benchmark current costs and current processes to document what happens after you make the staffing change. Internal benchmarking will permit a medical practice executive to demonstrate to the physicians that the change to staffing did in fact achieve the expected results.

4. *Should a practice develop a telephone nurse triage unit?*

Whether or not a practice elects to develop telephone nurse triage depends upon the type of inbound telephone calls that are currently received. If the majority of calls can be handled by nursing staff, nurse triage may be a valuable asset to the practice. In general pediatrics, for example, many practices have found that nurse triage assists in patient care management, with nurses following clinical protocols and providing parents with access to basic medical information, reducing unnecessary patient visits. At the same time, nurse triage permits the acuity of the patient to be triaged so that patients can be worked into the physician's schedule with priority during the day. From a financial perspective, the costs of nurse triage can be computed by identifying the current physician time devoted to these calls, the number of patient visits that did not need to occur if telephone triage was available, and the number of patient visits the physician could see if calls were first handled by nurse triage. If the practice elects to develop nurse triage support, these types of measures will permit the practice to analyze whether or not the addition of a telephone nurse triage unit had its intended effect.

5. *Why would a medical practice want to look at staffing per work relative value unit?*

Work relative value units are mapped to the CPT codes and essentially represent physician work effort. Physicians who practice with more complex cases or who perform more procedures will have higher work relative value units and may require a different staffing model to support this activity than their counterparts. Recognizing that staff is a measure of work, different staffing models to support physician work levels can be approached, such as changes to staffing skill mix, shared nursing functions, focused procedure staff, etc., to essentially match or rightsize staffing to the physician's work level.

Appendix II
Staffing Resource Allocation Tool

A tool to assist in the staff rightsizing process is provided in this Appendix. This tool incorporates both quantitative and qualitative measures to review a particular staff position in the medical practice for rightsizing opportunity. Appendix III and Appendix IV contain benchmarking data necessary to perform the quantitative analysis, and Appendix V contains staffing definitions consistent with the MGMA survey instruments.

STAFFING RESOURCE ALLOCATION TOOL

I. Position Reviewed: _____

II. General Duties and Responsibilities:

_____

_____

_____

_____

_____

III. Describe the Current Practice Model Involving this Position:

_____

_____

_____

IV. Describe the Current Staffing Model for this Work Function

General Administrative: _____

Business Office: _____

Patient Check-in: _____

Patient Check-out: _____

Clinical Support: _____

Telephone Management: _____

Medical Records: _____

Medical Transcription: _____

Ancillary: _____

Other: _____

V. Quantitative Staffing Analysis

TABLE 1 Overall Staffing Analysis

Staffing Analysis	Your Practice	MGMA* Peers	MGMA* Better Performers
Total Support Staff			
Support Staff Per FTE Physician			
Support Staff Per FTE Provider			
Support Staff Per CFTE Provider+			
Total Support Staff per 10,000 WRVU			
Total Support Staff per 10,000 Patients			
Total Support Staff per 10,000 Sq. Feet			
Staff Cost Per FTE Physician			
Staff Cost as % Total Medical Revenue			
Revenue After Total Operating Cost Per FTE Physician			

*Benchmarks provided in MGMA *Cost Survey Report*
**Benchmarks provided in MGMA *Performance and Practices of Successful Medical Groups Report*
+Calculate Clinical FTE equivalencies based on provider production data, e.g., WRVU

Conclusions

_____

_____

_____

TABLE 2 ■ FTE Staff per FTE Physician

Job Function	Your Practice	25th* Percentile	Median*	75th* Percentile
General Administrative				
Business Office				
Managed Care Administrative				
Information Technology				
Housekeeping, Maint., Security				
Medical Receptionists				
Med Secretaries, Transcribers				
Medical Records				
Other Administrative Support				
Registered Nurses				
Licensed Practical Nurses				
Medical Assistants, Nurse Aides				
Clinical Laboratory				
Radiology and Imaging				
Other Medical Support Services				
Total Employed Support Staff				
Total Contracted Support Staff				
Total Support Staff				

*Benchmarks Provided in Appendix III & Appendix IV of this text. (Select relevant specialty benchmark)

If not reported in the above figures for the medical group

FTE Equivalency for Overtime Incurred (Past One-Year Period)
_____ FTE

FTE Equivalency for Registry, Float, or Temporary Staff (Past One-Year Period)
_____ FTE

TABLE 3 ■ Categorical Staffing Analysis per FTE Physician

Staff Category	Your Practice	25th* Percentile	Median*	75th* Percentile
Administrative & Business Staff				
Front Office Staff				
Clinical Staff				
Ancillary Services Staff				

*Benchmarks Provided in Appendix III & Appendix IV of this text. (Select relevant specialty benchmark)

Conclusions

TABLE 4 ■ Staff Cost per FTE Physician

Job Function	Your Practice	25th* Percentile	Median*	75th* Percentile
General Administrative				
Business Office				
Managed Care Administrative				
Information Technology				
Housekeeping, Maint., Security				
Medical Receptionists				
Med Secretaries, Transcribers				
Medical Records				
Other Administrative Support				
Registered Nurses				
Licensed Practical Nurses				
Medical Assistants, Nurse Aides				
Clinical Laboratory				
Radiology and Imaging				
Other Medical Support Services				
Total Employed Support Staff				
Total Contracted Support Staff				
Total Support Staff				

*Benchmarks Provided in Appendix III & Appendix IV of this text. (Select relevant specialty benchmark)

TABLE 5 Categorical Staffing Cost per FTE Physician

Staff Category	Your Practice	25th* Percentile	Median*	75th* Percentile
Administrative & Business Staff				
Front Office Staff				
Clinical Staff				
Ancillary Services Staff				

*Benchmarks Provided in Appendix III & Appendix IV of this text. (Select relevant specialty benchmark)

Conclusions

_____

_____

_____

TABLE 6 ■ Staff Cost as a Percent of Total Medical Revenue

Job Function	Your Practice	25th* Percentile	Median*	75th* Percentile
General Administrative				
Business Office				
Managed Care Administrative				
Information Technology				
Housekeeping, Maint., Security				
Medical Receptionists				
Med Secretaries, Transcribers				
Medical Records				
Other Administrative Support				
Registered Nurses				
Licensed Practical Nurses				
Medical Assistants, Nurse Aides				
Clinical Laboratory				
Radiology and Imaging				
Other Medical Support Services				
Total Employed Support Staff				
Total Contracted Support Staff				
Total Support Staff				

*Benchmarks Provided in Appendix III & Appendix IV of this text. (Select relevant specialty benchmark)

TABLE 7 ■ Categorical Staff Cost Analysis As a Percent of Total Medical Revenue

Staff Category	Your Practice	25th* Percentile	Median*	75th* Percentile
Administrative & Business Staff				
Front Office Staff				
Clinical Staff				
Ancillary Services Staff				

*Benchmarks Provided in Appendix III & Appendix IV of this text. (Select relevant specialty benchmark)

Conclusions

_____

_____

_____

TABLE 8 ■ Performance Workload Ranges

Identify the workload of this position and compare it to the expected performance workload ranges established at the medical practice.

Work Process (Examples)	Performance Workload Range
Telephones with Message-Taking	
Appointment Scheduling with No Registration	
Appointment Scheduling with Full Registration	
Check-in with Registration Verification and Cashiering	
Nursing Support	
Nurse Triage	
Check-out with Scheduling, Charge Entry	
Referral Specialist	
Medical Records Chart Retrieval or Filing	
Medical Transcription	
Other	

Conclusions

_____

_____

_____

Summary of Conclusions from Quantitative Analysis

_____

_____

_____

_____

_____

VI. Qualitative Staffing Analysis

1. What is the potential for a change to the **practice model**?

2. What is the potential for a **shared staffing model** or performing the function with current staff through **workload redistribution**?

3. What is the potential for **centralizing versus distributing** this function?

4. What changes can be made in terms of **facility design or design of the practice site within the facility** that may permit staff savings and enhance practice efficiency?

5. What are the opportunities to **streamline this process,** such as reducing hand-offs, leveraging technology?

6. What are the other **internal, medical group specific factors** that may impact this position or create extenuating circumstances?

Appendix III
MGMA Benchmarks—
Peer Comparison Tables

106 ■ APPENDIX III

This Appendix provides the key staffing benchmarks to be used in Step 1—Benchmark the Current State, when comparing a practice's staffing to those of its peers. The data include benchmarks at the **staff category level** (front office staff, general and administrative staff, clinical support staff, and ancillary service staff) as well as the **staff job classification level** for 28 different specialties and group practice ownership categories.

The following tables are computed from the Medical Group Management Association (MGMA) *Cost Survey: 2001 Report Based on 2000 Data.* The Cost Survey Report summarizes the financial performance and productivity of responding medical practices and presents a comprehensive fiscal picture of medical group practice. In addition to the staffing ratios reported below, the Cost Survey reports medical revenue, staff salary costs, total operating costs, revenue after operating costs, provider cost, and net practice income/loss. Accounts receivable, payer mix, collection percentages, financial ratios and balance sheet information are also reported.

The MGMA *Cost Survey: 2001 Report Based on 2000 Data* database consists of data provided by 1,161 medical group practices. Participation in the survey is voluntary, and participants were not compensated for their participation. The survey is primarily a survey of MGMA members, and MGMA does not claim that the results are necessarily representative of the national medical practice population.

Each table has four statistics:

1. count
2. 25th percentile (abbreviated in the table as 25th %tile)
3. median
4. 75th percentile (abbreviated in the table as 75th %tile).

The count is the number of medical practices reporting staffing for the table. The 25th percentile is that point in a frequency distribution arranged from lowest to highest where one-fourth (25 percent) of the values are less. The median is the midpoint of all responses, and the 75th percentile is the point where three-fourths (75 percent) are less. When an * appears in the table, an insufficient number of responses were received to compute and report that data element.

In examining the data presented in this Appendix, the medical practice executive might want to consider the following:

The range of values between the 25th percentile and the 75th percentile includes half of the responses and is considered the range of normal responses. Conversely, if the practice's staffing is either above the 75th percentile or less than the 25th percentile of similar types of practices, further examination may be appropriate. The practice executive should ask:

1. Is the comparison made to a similar type of medical practice? Staffing will vary considerably by type of practice and comparisons should be made to the practice type that is most similar to the medical group (by specialty and whether or not the practice is owned by a hospital or by physicians).
2. What is the difference between the data reported by the practice and the 25th percentile (if lower) or 75th percentile (if greater)?

3. Do these differences indicate that the practice's performance is significantly out of line with the cost survey statistics? Such differences may help identify some areas of the practice's business that require closer scrutiny.
4. Are the differences explainable either through the practice's method of data collection, data reporting and/or data definitions, or because of special practice goals?
5. By what methods can staffing be changed or managed?

TABLE 1 ■ All Multispecialty Practices

Table 1a. FTE Staff per FTE Physician

	All Multispecialty Groups			
	Count	**25th %tile**	**Median**	**75th %tile**
General administrative	296	0.17	0.25	0.36
Business office	300	0.50	0.72	0.97
Managed care administrative	109	0.03	0.10	0.21
Information technology	165	0.06	0.10	0.17
Housekeeping, maintenance, security	169	0.04	0.11	0.21
Medical receptionists	290	0.64	0.88	1.18
Med secretaries, transcribers	246	0.14	0.25	0.41
Medical records	264	0.25	0.38	0.54
Other administrative support	157	0.06	0.14	0.38
Registered nurses	269	0.23	0.49	0.80
Licensed practical nurses	264	0.21	0.46	0.82
Medical assistants, nurse aides	274	0.35	0.61	0.91
Clinical laboratory	240	0.20	0.32	0.46
Radiology and imaging	239	0.12	0.21	0.34
Other medical support services	167	0.09	0.23	0.44
Total employed support staff	329	4.00	4.92	5.83
Total contracted support staff	128	0.06	0.14	0.26
Total support staff	333	4.05	4.96	5.93

Table 1b. Staff Cost per FTE Physician

	All Multispecialty Groups			
	Count	**25th %tile**	**Median**	**75th %tile**
General administrative	296	$10,010	$14,292	$19,545
Business office	301	$13,013	$17,379	$23,159
Managed care administrative	111	$1,150	$2,803	$6,612
Information technology	166	$2,021	$3,539	$5,207
Housekeeping, maintenance, security	174	$966	$2,555	$4,369
Medical receptionists	288	$11,606	$16,929	$23,626
Medical secretaries, transcribers	248	$3,295	$5,891	$9,840
Medical records	260	$4,380	$6,783	$9,903
Other administrative support	164	$952	$3,110	$8,527
Registered nurses	268	$8,752	$16,143	$28,377
Licensed practical nurses	265	$6,189	$11,932	$19,441
Medical assistants, nurse aides	273	$6,856	$12,266	$19,005
Clinical laboratory	239	$5,766	$8,959	$12,113
Radiology and imaging	239	$3,629	$6,702	$11,578
Other medical support services	172	$3,185	$6,446	$13,632
Total employed support staff cost	332	$101,785	$126,931	$153,804
Total employed support staff benefits	321	$19,689	$28,397	$37,461
Total contracted support staff	186	$2,175	$4,614	$8,846
Total support staff cost	333	$126,353	$156,492	$194,441

TABLE 1 Continued

Table 1c. Staff Cost As a Percent of Total Medical Revenue

		All Multispecialty Groups		
	Count	25th %tile	Median	75th %tile
General administrative	296	1.96%	2.62%	3.79%
Business office	301	2.60%	3.34%	4.36%
Managed care administrative	111	0.26%	0.59%	1.18%
Information technology	166	0.38%	0.58%	0.90%
Housekeeping, maintenance, security	174	0.19%	0.44%	0.71%
Medical receptionists	288	2.03%	3.16%	5.00%
Medical secretaries, transcribers	248	0.63%	1.22%	1.75%
Medical records	260	0.83%	1.22%	1.88%
Other administrative support	164	0.16%	0.59%	1.79%
Registered nurses	268	1.65%	3.09%	5.35%
Licensed practical nurses	265	1.22%	2.15%	4.01%
Medical assistants, nurse aides	273	1.30%	2.44%	3.81%
Clinical laboratory	239	1.03%	1.54%	2.18%
Radiology and imaging	239	0.76%	1.28%	1.88%
Other medical support services	172	0.58%	1.20%	2.11%
Total employed support staff cost	332	21.35%	25.06%	30.58%
Total employed support staff benefits	321	4.44%	5.56%	6.80%
Total contracted support staff	186	0.40%	0.92%	1.55%
Total support staff cost	333	26.57%	31.20%	37.46%

Table 1d. FTE Staff per FTE Physician (Staff Categories)

		All Multispecialty Groups		
	Count	25th %tile	Median	75th %tile
Administrative and Business Staff per FTE Physician	313	0.80	1.17	1.52
Front Office Staff per FTE Physician	312	1.24	1.59	1.97
Clinical Staff per FTE Physician	306	1.26	1.50	1.84
Ancillary Service Staff per FTE Physician	278	0.36	0.66	1.02

Table 1e. Staff Cost Per FTE Physician (Staff Categories)

		All Multispecialty Groups		
	Count	25th %tile	Median	75th %tile
Administrative and Business Staff Salary per FTE Physician	312	$27,022	$36,223	$46,554
Front Office Staff Salary per FTE Physician	310	$24,508	$31,638	$39,649
Clinical Staff Salary per FTE Physician	306	$31,404	$40,701	$52,072
Ancillary Service Staff Salary per FTE Physician	279	$9,000	$19,325	$30,483

Table 1f. Staff Cost As a Percent of Total Medical Revenue (Staff Categories)

		All Multispecialty Groups		
	Count	25th %tile	Median	75th %tile
Administrative and Business Staff Salary As % of Total Medical Revenue	312	5.41%	7.09%	8.86%
Front Office Staff Salary As % of Total Medical Revenue	310	4.66%	6.17%	8.26%
Clinical Staff Salary As % of Total Medical Revenue	306	6.23%	7.96%	10.35%
Ancillary Service Staff Salary As % of Total Medical Revenue	279	2.23%	3.61%	4.97%

TABLE 2 ■ Multispecialty Practices, Not Hospital/Integrated Delivery System Owned

Table 2a. FTE Staff per FTE Physician

Multispecialty Not Hospital Owned

	Count	25th %tile	Median	75th %tile
General administrative	211	0.18	0.25	0.35
Business office	212	0.57	0.76	0.97
Managed care administrative	75	0.04	0.10	0.23
Information technology	134	0.07	0.11	0.19
Housekeeping, maintenace, security	134	0.06	0.13	0.22
Medical receptionists	205	0.62	0.83	1.15
Medical secretaries, transcribers	177	0.15	0.28	0.44
Medical records	196	0.27	0.40	0.55
Other administrative support	106	0.05	0.10	0.23
Registered nurses	187	0.23	0.49	0.79
Licensed practical nurses	177	0.21	0.46	0.82
Medical assistants, nurse aides	187	0.38	0.63	0.94
Clinical laboratory	183	0.23	0.34	0.48
Radiology and imaging	174	0.15	0.25	0.37
Other medical support services	127	0.11	0.25	0.45
Total employed support staff	220	4.24	5.16	6.12
Total contracted support staff	93	0.06	0.14	0.26
Total support staff	222	4.35	5.19	6.28

Table 2b. Staff Cost per FTE Physician

Multispecialty Not Hospital Owned

	Count	25th %tile	Median	75th %tile
General administrative	212	$9,993	$14,111	$18,786
Business office	214	$14,552	$17,819	$23,410
Managed care administrative	77	$1,395	$3,521	$7,331
Information technology	135	$2,230	$3,702	$5,354
Housekeeping, maintenance, security	139	$1,359	$2,916	$4,487
Medical receptionists	206	$11,574	$16,717	$22,411
Medical secretaries, transcribers	179	$3,694	$6,334	$10,272
Medical records	195	$4,659	$7,066	$9,945
Other administrative support	111	$923	$1,954	$5,045
Registered nurses	187	$8,885	$15,531	$28,089
Licensed practical nurses	179	$6,166	$11,946	$19,500
Medical assistants, nurse aides	188	$7,613	$13,145	$19,693
Clinical laboratory	184	$6,891	$9,512	$12,336
Radiology and imaging	176	$4,336	$7,853	$12,035
Other medical support services	131	$3,471	$7,182	$13,659
Total employed support staff cost	221	$107,155	$134,251	$164,270
Total employed support staff benefits	214	$22,299	$30,353	$40,606
Total contracted support staff	130	$1,984	$4,162	$7,585
Total support staff cost	222	$133,680	$166,978	$206,602

TABLE 2 ■ Continued

Table 2c. Staff Cost As a Percent of Total Medical Revenue

Multispecialty Not Hospital Owned

	Count	25th %tile	Median	75th %tile
General administrative	212	1.82%	2.37%	3.45%
Business office	214	2.60%	3.20%	4.09%
Managed care administrative	77	0.24%	0.62%	1.23%
Information technology	135	0.38%	0.57%	0.89%
Housekeeping, maintenance, security	139	0.24%	0.49%	0.73%
Medical receptionists	206	1.93%	2.75%	4.41%
Medical secretaries, transcribers	179	0.66%	1.23%	1.63%
Medical records	195	0.81%	1.19%	1.77%
Other administrative support	111	0.14%	0.38%	1.08%
Registered nurses	187	1.45%	2.60%	4.69%
Licensed practical nurses	179	1.12%	1.88%	3.68%
Medical assistants, nurse aides	188	1.22%	2.36%	3.59%
Clinical laboratory	184	1.15%	1.64%	2.17%
Radiology and imaging	176	0.76%	1.32%	1.92%
Other medical support services	131	0.62%	1.22%	2.09%
Total employed support staff cost	221	20.81%	23.94%	27.56%
Total employed support staff benefits	214	4.33%	5.49%	6.58%
Total contracted support staff	130	0.37%	0.73%	1.35%
Total support staff cost	222	26.14%	29.41%	34.38%

Table 2d. FTE Staff per FTE Physician (Staff Categories)

Multispecialty Not Hospital Owned

	Count	25th %tile	Median	75th %tile
Administrative and Business Staff per FTE Physician	215	0.99	1.26	1.59
Front Office Staff per FTE Physician	213	1.26	1.61	1.95
Clinical Staff per FTE Physician	209	1.26	1.50	1.84
Ancillary Service Staff per FTE Physician	200	0.48	0.75	1.11

Table 2e. Staff Cost per FTE Physician (Staff Categories)

Multispecialty Not Hospital Owned

	Count	25th %tile	Median	75th %tile
Administrative and Business Staff Salary per FTE Physician	216	$ 29,910	$ 39,007	$ 49,803
Front Office Staff Salary per FTE Physician	214	$ 25,642	$ 31,794	$ 39,828
Clinical Staff Salary per FTE Physician	210	$ 31,360	$ 42,074	$ 52,072
Ancillary Service Staff Salary per FTE Physician	202	$ 13,312	$ 22,372	$ 32,682

Table 2f. Staff Cost As a Percent of Total Medical Revenue (Staff Categories)

Multispecialty Not Hospital Owned

	Count	25th %tile	Median	75th %tile
Front Office Staff Salary As % of Total Medical Revenue	214	4.45%	5.73%	7.58%
Admin and Business Staff Salary As % of Total Medical Revenue	216	5.51%	6.79%	8.36%
Clinical Staff Salary As % of Total Medical Revenue	210	5.79%	7.19%	9.08%
Ancillary Service Staff Salary As % of Total Medical Revenue	202	2.60%	3.86%	4.97%

TABLE 3 — Multispecialty, Hospital/Integrated Delivery System Owned

Table 3a. FTE Staff per FTE Physician

	Multispecialty (Hospital / IDS Owned)			
	Count	**25th %tile**	**Median**	**75th %tile**
General administrative	85	0.17	0.27	0.41
Business office	88	0.35	0.62	0.91
Managed care administrative	34	0.03	0.09	0.17
Information technology	31	0.04	0.07	0.12
Housekeeping, maintenance, security	35	0.02	0.04	0.12
Medical receptionists	85	0.67	0.96	1.25
Medical secretaries, transcribers	69	0.09	0.20	0.38
Medical records	68	0.16	0.33	0.49
Other administrative support	51	0.09	0.33	1.19
Registered nurses	82	0.20	0.49	0.95
Licensed practical nurses	87	0.23	0.46	0.80
Medical assistants, nurse aides	87	0.28	0.52	0.78
Clinical laboratory	57	0.09	0.25	0.35
Radiology and imaging	65	0.10	0.16	0.23
Other medical support services	40	0.05	0.12	0.36
Total employed support staff	109	3.37	4.45	5.22
Total contracted support staff	35	0.07	0.14	0.33
Total support staff	111	3.42	4.47	5.38

Table 3b. Staff Cost per FTE Physician

	Multispecialty (Hospital / IDS Owned)			
	Count	**25th %tile**	**Median**	**75th %tile**
General administrative	84	$10,058	$14,667	$21,421
Business office	87	$9,069	$13,754	$22,343
Managed care administrative	34	$992	$2,038	$4,613
Information technology	31	$1,605	$2,807	$4,211
Housekeeping, maintenance, security	35	$490	$966	$2,428
Medical receptionists	82	$11,668	$18,434	$24,943
Medical secretaries, transcribers	69	$2,535	$4,862	$8,012
Medical records	65	$3,172	$5,598	$8,747
Other administrative support	53	$2,270	$7,580	$20,742
Registered nurses	81	$8,322	$18,030	$29,876
Licensed practical nurses	86	$6,211	$11,931	$19,399
Medical assistants, nurse aides	85	$6,381	$10,664	$17,652
Clinical laboratory	55	$1,930	$6,669	$9,720
Radiology and imaging	63	$2,494	$4,544	$7,977
Other medical support services	41	$1,347	$4,491	$12,738
Total employed support staff cost	111	$86,407	$114,255	$135,655
Total employed support staff benefits	107	$16,758	$22,418	$31,510
Total contracted support staff	56	$2,251	$5,229	$10,774
Total support staff cost	111	$108,778	$142,673	$167,575

TABLE 3 ■ Continued

Table 3c. Staff Cost As a Percent of Total Medical Revenue

	Multispecialty (Hospital / IDS Owned)			
	Count	25th %tile	Median	75th %tile
General administrative	84	2.46%	3.65%	5.41%
Business office	87	2.60%	3.70%	5.29%
Managed care administrative	34	0.25%	0.59%	1.02%
Information technology	31	0.37%	0.61%	0.93%
Housekeeping, maintenance, security	35	0.12%	0.20%	0.55%
Medical receptionists	82	2.71%	4.75%	6.91%
Medical secretaries, transcribers	69	0.61%	1.14%	2.00%
Medical records	65	0.84%	1.32%	2.37%
Other administrative support	53	0.58%	2.04%	5.33%
Registered nurses	81	2.09%	4.43%	7.97%
Licensed practical nurses	86	1.59%	2.95%	5.31%
Medical assistants, nurse aides	85	1.48%	2.89%	4.59%
Clinical laboratory	55	0.50%	1.30%	2.30%
Radiology and imaging	63	0.72%	1.14%	1.63%
Other medical support services	41	0.39%	1.18%	2.48%
Total employed support staff cost	111	23.23%	28.79%	34.19%
Total employed support staff benefits	107	4.82%	5.97%	7.49%
Total contracted support staff	56	0.56%	1.12%	2.63%
Total support staff cost	111	29.57%	35.68%	42.09%

Table 3d. FTE Staff per FTE Physician (Staff Categories)

	Multispecialty (Hospital / IDS Owned)			
	Count	25th %tile	Median	75th %tile
Administrative and Business Staff per FTE Physician	98	0.45	0.90	1.27
Front Office Staff per FTE Physician	99	1.21	1.55	2.00
Clinical Staff per FTE Physician	97	1.19	1.50	1.93
Ancillary Service Staff per FTE Physician	78	0.18	0.40	0.74

Table 3e. Staff Cost per FTE Physician (Staff Categories)

	Multispecialty (Hospital / IDS Owned)			
	Count	25th %tile	Median	75th %tile
Administrative and Business Staff Salary per FTE Physician	96	$ 18,001	$ 31,393	$ 41,183
Front Office Staff Salary per FTE Physician	96	$ 21,978	$ 31,407	$ 38,955
Clinical Staff Salary per FTE Physician	96	$ 31,668	$ 39,840	$ 52,325
Ancillary Service Staff Salary per FTE Physician	77	$ 5,805	$ 13,043	$ 22,533

Table 3f. Staff Cost As a Percent of Total Medical Revenue (Staff Categories)

	Multispecialty (Hospital / IDS Owned)			
	Count	25th %tile	Median	75th %tile
Administrative and Business Staff Salary As % of Total Medical Revenue	96	4.83%	7.80%	10.60%
Front Office Staff Salary As % of Total Medical Revenue	96	5.59%	7.98%	11.10%
Clinical Staff Salary As % of Total Medical Revenue	96	8.02%	10.44%	12.97%
Ancillary Service Staff Salary As % of Total Medical Revenue	77	1.43%	2.95%	4.88%

TABLE 4 — Multispecialty with Primary Care Only, Not Hospital/Integrated Delivery System Owned

Table 4a. FTE Staff per FTE Physician

Multispecialty with Primary Care Only (Not Hospital / IDS Owned)

	Count	25th %tile	Median	75th %tile
General administrative	41	0.13	0.25	0.44
Business office	41	0.50	0.71	0.98
Managed care administrative	9	*	*	*
Information technology	12	0.04	0.11	0.15
Housekeeping, maintenance, security	21	0.05	0.14	0.31
Medical receptionists	40	0.75	1.16	1.39
Medical secretaries, transcribers	31	0.14	0.29	0.49
Medical records	33	0.22	0.31	0.49
Other administrative support	11	0.07	0.18	0.25
Registered nurses	33	0.20	0.44	0.72
Licensed practical nurses	37	0.24	0.50	1.06
Medical assistants, nurse aides	38	0.43	0.74	1.05
Clinical laboratory	33	0.24	0.37	0.67
Radiology and imaging	25	0.13	0.23	0.44
Other medical support services	11	0.11	0.20	0.42
Total employed support staff	44	3.98	4.94	6.41
Total contracted support staff	19	0.08	0.24	0.30
Total support staff	44	4.09	5.00	6.61

Table 4b. Staff Cost per FTE Physician

Multispecialty with Primary Care Only (Not Hospital / IDS Owned)

	Count	25th %tile	Median	75th %tile
General administrative	42	$ 9,697	$ 13,708	$ 23,988
Business office	42	$ 12,224	$ 17,252	$ 23,108
Managed care administrative	10	$ 2,966	$ 5,458	$ 15,352
Information technology	12	$ 1,694	$ 3,716	$ 4,495
Housekeeping, maintenance, security	21	$ 997	$ 2,978	$ 5,228
Medical receptionists	40	$ 13,174	$ 20,448	$ 26,483
Medical secretaries, transcribers	32	$ 3,364	$ 6,195	$ 9,143
Medical records	33	$ 3,889	$ 5,000	$ 8,991
Other administrative support	12	$ 1,491	$ 4,362	$ 6,028
Registered nurses	33	$ 4,469	$ 13,010	$ 24,778
Licensed practical nurses	37	$ 6,494	$ 10,991	$ 24,853
Medical assistants, nurse aides	38	$ 8,492	$ 13,704	$ 22,034
Clinical laboratory	33	$ 6,489	$ 9,835	$ 15,854
Radiology and imaging	26	$ 3,276	$ 6,358	$ 11,864
Other medical support services	13	$ 2,760	$ 3,471	$ 8,666
Total employed support staff cost	44	$ 93,962	$ 123,979	$ 157,944
Total employed support staff benefits	43	$ 19,684	$ 25,615	$ 35,307
Total contracted support staff	23	$ 1,578	$ 4,829	$ 7,639
Total support staff cost	44	$ 130,474	$ 149,880	$ 191,353

TABLE 4 — Continued

Table 4c. Staff Cost As a Percent of Total Medical Revenue

	\multicolumn{4}{c}{Multispecialty with Primary Care Only (Not Hospital / IDS Owned)}
	Count	25th %tile	Median	75th %tile
General administrative	42	1.98%	2.97%	4.38%
Business office	42	2.87%	3.52%	4.86%
Managed care administrative	10	0.69%	1.23%	2.39%
Information technology	12	0.38%	0.65%	0.98%
Housekeeping, maintenance, security	21	0.26%	0.52%	0.99%
Medical receptionists	40	2.57%	3.93%	5.75%
Medical secretaries, transcribers	32	0.72%	1.16%	2.00%
Medical records	33	0.74%	1.07%	1.54%
Other administrative support	12	0.33%	0.74%	1.21%
Registered nurses	33	0.94%	2.47%	5.19%
Licensed practical nurses	37	1.24%	2.90%	4.11%
Medical assistants, nurse aides	38	1.58%	2.90%	5.33%
Clinical laboratory	33	1.37%	1.90%	3.05%
Radiology and imaging	26	0.73%	1.31%	2.04%
Other medical support services	13	0.44%	0.69%	1.37%
Total employed support staff cost	44	21.22%	25.01%	30.09%
Total employed support staff benefits	43	4.46%	5.51%	6.54%
Total contracted support staff	23	0.43%	0.97%	1.54%
Total support staff cost	44	27.85%	29.98%	37.18%

Table 4d. FTE Staff per FTE Physician (Staff Categories)

	\multicolumn{4}{c}{Multispecialty with Primary Care Only (Not Hospital / IDS Owned)}
	Count	25th %tile	Median	75th %tile
Administrative and Business Staff per FTE Physician	41	1.31	1.61	1.94
Front Office Staff per FTE Physician	43	0.74	1.06	1.76
Clinical Staff per FTE Physician	42	1.26	1.75	2.05
Ancillary Service Staff per FTE Physician	37	0.27	0.56	1.04

Table 4e. Staff Cost per FTE Physician (Staff Categories)

	\multicolumn{4}{c}{Multispecialty with Primary Care Only (Not Hospital / IDS Owned)}
	Count	25th %tile	Median	75th %tile
Administrative and Business Staff Salary per FTE Physician	41	$25,676	$32,035	$35,948
Front Office Staff Salary per FTE Physician	43	$24,233	$33,052	$60,380
Clinical Staff Salary per FTE Physician	42	$29,280	$43,695	$54,429
Ancillary Service Staff Salary per FTE Physician	37	$7,227	$13,839	$28,699

Table 4f. Staff Cost As a Percent of Total Medical Revenue (Staff Categories)

	\multicolumn{4}{c}{Multispecialty with Primary Care Only (Not Hospital / IDS Owned)}
	Count	25th %tile	Median	75th %tile
Administrative and Business Staff Salary As % of Total Medical Revenue	41	4.82%	6.53%	8.31%
Front Office Staff Salary As % of Total Medical Revenue	43	5.11%	7.42%	9.79%
Clinical Staff Salary As % of Total Medical Revenue	42	6.30%	8.46%	10.55%
Ancillary Service Staff Salary As % of Total Medical Revenue	37	1.49%	3.10%	4.60%

TABLE 5 ■ Multispecialty with Primary Care Only, Hospital/Integrated Delivery System Owned

Table 5a. FTE Staff per FTE Physician

Multispecialty with Primary Care Only (Hospital / IDS Owned)

	Count	25th %tile	Median	75th %tile
General administrative	38	0.19	0.30	0.41
Business office	40	0.28	0.49	0.89
Managed care administrative	14	0.03	0.10	0.17
Information technology	13	0.04	0.07	0.12
Housekeeping, maintenance, security	11	0.02	0.05	0.11
Medical receptionists	41	0.75	1.03	1.39
Medical secretaries, transcribers	29	0.09	0.19	0.40
Medical records	33	0.14	0.29	0.53
Other administrative support	22	0.11	0.39	1.37
Registered nurses	36	0.30	0.73	1.27
Licensed practical nurses	42	0.24	0.41	0.91
Medical assistants, nurse aides	41	0.32	0.61	0.94
Clinical laboratory	24	0.07	0.26	0.33
Radiology and imaging	29	0.10	0.15	0.22
Other medical support services	13	0.02	0.13	0.59
Total employed support staff	53	3.43	4.47	5.22
Total contracted support staff	17	0.06	0.14	0.27
Total support staff	54	3.45	4.48	5.30

Table 5b. Staff Cost per FTE Physician

Multispecialty with Primary Care Only (Hospital / IDS Owned)

	Count	25th %tile	Median	75th %tile
General administrative	37	$ 11,260	$ 15,451	$ 21,572
Business office	39	$ 8,126	$ 12,512	$ 24,981
Managed care administrative	14	$ 1,490	$ 2,736	$ 5,719
Information technology	13	$ 1,632	$ 2,955	$ 4,590
Housekeeping, maintenance, security	10	$ 312	$ 1,082	$ 4,237
Medical receptionists	37	$ 14,501	$ 20,933	$ 26,613
Medical secretaries, transcribers	28	$ 1,762	$ 5,327	$ 8,026
Medical records	30	$ 2,418	$ 5,269	$ 9,765
Other administrative support	23	$ 2,335	$ 9,983	$ 30,377
Registered nurses	34	$ 9,568	$ 26,337	$ 38,144
Licensed practical nurses	40	$ 6,304	$ 10,064	$ 22,615
Medical assistants, nurse aides	38	$ 6,784	$ 11,136	$ 23,916
Clinical laboratory	22	$ 1,352	$ 7,593	$ 10,268
Radiology and imaging	27	$ 2,812	$ 4,281	$ 6,702
Other medical support services	14	$ 903	$ 5,519	$ 12,471
Total employed support staff cost	54	$ 86,382	$ 117,769	$ 135,991
Total employed support staff benefits	53	$ 16,608	$ 22,418	$ 29,921
Total contracted support staff	26	$ 2,159	$ 4,867	$ 9,782
Total support staff cost	54	$ 107,629	$ 144,623	$ 172,315

TABLE 5 — Continued

Table 5c. Staff Cost As a Percent of Total Medical Revenue

Multispecialty with Primary Care Only (Hospital / IDS Owned)

	Count	25th %tile	Median	75th %tile
General administrative	37	3.36%	4.19%	5.69%
Business office	39	2.77%	3.88%	5.59%
Managed care administrative	14	0.44%	0.69%	1.34%
Information technology	13	0.41%	0.61%	1.24%
Housekeeping, maintenance, security	10	0.08%	0.30%	0.66%
Medical receptionists	37	3.36%	6.09%	7.45%
Medical secretaries, transcribers	28	0.58%	1.47%	2.08%
Medical records	30	0.82%	1.46%	2.42%
Other administrative support	23	0.59%	2.56%	10.99%
Registered nurses	34	2.22%	7.14%	11.19%
Licensed practical nurses	40	1.76%	3.00%	6.99%
Medical assistants, nurse aides	38	2.07%	3.23%	5.55%
Clinical laboratory	22	0.40%	1.41%	2.60%
Radiology and imaging	27	0.93%	1.14%	1.57%
Other medical support services	14	0.21%	1.35%	3.96%
Total employed support staff cost	54	26.01%	31.55%	35.70%
Total employed support staff benefits	53	5.17%	6.54%	7.96%
Total contracted support staff	26	0.55%	1.12%	3.07%
Total support staff cost	54	33.01%	39.69%	44.93%

Table 5d. FTE Staff per FTE Physician (Staff Categories)

Multispecialty with Primary Care Only (Hospital / IDS Owned)

	Count	25th %tile	Median	75th %tile
Administrative and Business Staff per FTE Physician	45	0.40	0.76	1.22
Front Office Staff per FTE Physician	48	1.25	1.59	2.10
Clinical Staff per FTE Physician	47	1.36	1.64	2.12
Ancillary Service Staff per FTE Physician	34	0.15	0.34	0.62

Table 5e. Staff Cost per FTE Physician (Staff Categories)

Multispecialty Groups with Primary Care Only, Hospital / IDS Owned)

	Count	25th %tile	Median	75th %tile
Administrative and Business Staff Salary per FTE Physician	43	$18,072	$30,148	$44,807
Front Office Staff Salary per FTE Physician	45	$23,594	$31,851	$42,559
Clinical Staff Salary per FTE Physician	45	$31,918	$42,862	$56,813
Ancillary Service Staff Salary per FTE Physician	33	$3,911	$9,224	$17,774

Table 5f. Staff Cost As a Percent of Total Medical Revenue (Staff Categories)

Multispecialty with Primary Care Only (Hospital / IDS Owned)

	Count	25th %tile	Median	75th %tile
Administrative and Business Staff Salary As % of Total Medical Revenue	43	5.43%	8.41%	11.19%
Front Office Staff Salary As % of Total Medical Revenue	45	7.08%	9.06%	12.18%
Clinical Staff Salary As % of Total Medical Revenue	45	9.40%	11.91%	15.25%
Ancillary Service Staff Salary As % of Total Medical Revenue	33	1.19%	2.56%	4.88%

TABLE 6 ■ Allergy/Immunology, Not Hospital/Integrated Delivery System Owned

Table 6a. FTE Staff per FTE Physician

		Allergy / Immunology		
	Count	25th %tile	Median	75th %tile
General administrative	6	*	*	*
Business office	10	0.57	0.83	1.68
Managed care administrative	2	*	*	*
Information technology	1	*	*	*
Housekeeping, maintenance, security	3	*	*	*
Medical receptionists	10	0.75	1.23	1.51
Medical secretaries, transcribers	9	*	*	*
Medical records	3	*	*	*
Other administrative support	3	*	*	*
Registered nurses	8	*	*	*
Licensed practical nurses	9	*	*	*
Medical assistants, nurse aides	6	*	*	*
Clinical laboratory	5	*	*	*
Radiology and imaging	0	*	*	*
Other medical support services	1	*	*	*
Total employed support staff	11	4.10	4.88	7.06
Total contracted support staff	1	*	*	*
Total support staff	11	4.10	5.13	7.06

Table 6b. Staff Cost per FTE Physician

		Allergy / Immunology		
	Count	25th %tile	Median	75th %tile
General administrative	6	*	*	*
Business office	10	$ 14,038	$ 25,238	$ 40,532
Managed care administrative	2	*	*	*
Information technology	1	*	*	*
Housekeeping, maintenance, security	3	*	*	*
Medical receptionists	10	$ 12,077	$ 23,396	$ 34,173
Medical secretaries, transcribers	9	*	*	*
Medical records	3	*	*	*
Other administrative support	3	*	*	*
Registered nurses	7	*	*	*
Licensed practical nurses	9	*	*	*
Medical assistants, nurse aides	5	*	*	*
Clinical laboratory	5	*	*	*
Radiology and imaging	0	*	*	*
Other medical support services	1	*	*	*
Total employed support staff cost	11	$ 104,258	$ 128,001	$ 194,000
Total employed support staff benefits	11	$ 22,094	$ 29,000	$ 41,993
Total contracted support staff	2	*	*	*
Total support staff cost	11	$ 126,302	$ 161,466	$ 222,870

TABLE 6 ■ Continued

Table 6c. Staff Cost As a Percent of Total Medical Revenue

	Count	Allergy / Immunology 25th %tile	Median	75th %tile
General administrative	6	*	*	*
Business office	10	2.48%	4.24%	5.14%
Managed care administrative	2	*	*	*
Information technology	1	*	*	*
Housekeeping, maintenance, security	3	*	*	*
Medical receptionists	10	2.27%	3.21%	4.42%
Medical secretaries, transcribers	9	*	*	*
Medical records	3	*	*	*
Other administrative support	3	*	*	*
Registered nurses	7	*	*	*
Licensed practical nurses	9	*	*	*
Medical assistants, nurse aides	5	*	*	*
Clinical laboratory	5	*	*	*
Radiology and imaging	0	*	*	*
Other medical support services	1	*	*	*
Total employed support staff cost	11	17.77%	20.51%	22.70%
Total employed support staff benefits	11	4.04%	4.85%	6.84%
Total contracted support staff	2	*	*	*
Total support staff cost	11	21.90%	26.83%	29.41%

Table 6d. FTE Staff per FTE Physician (Staff Categories)

	Count	Allergy / Immunology 25th %tile	Median	75th %tile
Administrative and Business Staff per FTE Physician	10	0.80	1.20	1.86
Front Office Staff per FTE Physician	10	1.16	1.51	1.84
Clinical Staff per FTE Physician	10	1.86	2.10	3.03
Ancillary Service Staff per FTE Physician	6	*	*	*

Table 6e. Staff Cost per FTE Physician (Staff Categories)

	Count	Allergy / Immunology 25th %tile	Median	75th %tile
Administrative and Business Staff Salary per FTE Physician	10	$ 28,653	$ 41,534	$ 49,112
Front Office Staff Salary per FTE Physician	10	$ 16,341	$ 32,612	$ 43,400
Clinical Staff Salary per FTE Physician	10	$ 38,460	$ 42,808	$ 86,417
Ancillary Service Staff Salary per FTE Physician	6	*	*	*

Table 6f. Staff Cost As a Percent of Total Medical Revenue (Staff Categories)

	Count	Allergy / Immunology 25th %tile	Median	75th %tile
Front Office Staff Salary As % of Total Medical Revenue	10	2.62%	4.14%	6.54%
Administrative and Business Staff Salary As % of Total Medical Revenue	10	4.66%	6.11%	7.07%
Clinical Staff Salary As % of Total Medical Revenue	10	7.06%	7.91%	10.43%
Ancillary Service Staff Salary As % of Total Medical Revenue	6	*	*	*

TABLE 7 ■ Anesthesiology, Not Hospital/Integrated Delivery System Owned

Table 7a. FTE Staff per FTE Physician

	Count	25th %tile	Median	75th %tile
General administrative	36	0.04	0.06	0.08
Business office	38	0.27	0.33	0.59
Managed care administrative	1	*	*	*
Information technology	4	*	*	*
Housekeeping, maintenance, security	1	*	*	*
Medical receptionists	7	*	*	*
Medical secretaries, transcribers	10	0.05	0.07	0.12
Medical records	2	*	*	*
Other administrative support	6	*	*	*
Registered nurses	10	0.04	0.09	0.22
Licensed practical nurses	2	*	*	*
Medical assistants, nurse aides	3	*	*	*
Clinical laboratory	0	*	*	*
Radiology and imaging	0	*	*	*
Other medical support services	1	*	*	*
Total employed support staff	43	0.29	0.42	0.72
Total contracted support staff	4	*	*	*
Total support staff	45	0.30	0.42	0.74

Table 7b. Staff Cost per FTE Physician

	Count	25th %tile	Median	75th %tile
General administrative	36	$ 3,967	$ 5,204	$ 7,282
Business office	38	$ 7,712	$ 9,848	$ 17,294
Managed care administrative	1	*	*	*
Information technology	4	*	*	*
Housekeeping, maintenance, security	2	*	*	*
Medical receptionists	7	*	*	*
Medical secretaries, transcribers	10	$ 1,606	$ 1,903	$ 3,121
Medical records	2	*	*	*
Other administrative support	6	*	*	*
Registered nurses	10	$ 1,812	$ 4,118	$ 10,182
Licensed practical nurses	2	*	*	*
Medical assistants, nurse aides	3	*	*	*
Clinical laboratory	0	*	*	*
Radiology and imaging	0	*	*	*
Other medical support services	1	*	*	*
Total employed support staff cost	44	$ 10,303	$ 16,974	$ 25,815
Total employed support staff benefits	0	$ 3,240	$ 5,272	$ 7,085
Total contracted support staff	7	*	*	*
Total support staff cost	45	$ 14,119	$ 22,732	$ 31,378

TABLE 7 Continued

Table 7c. Staff Cost As a Percent of Total Medical Revenue

	Anesthesiology			
	Count	25th %tile	Median	75th %tile
General administrative	36	0.84%	1.17%	1.42%
Business office	38	1.45%	2.10%	3.28%
Managed care administrative	1	*	*	*
Information technology	4	*	*	*
Housekeeping, maintenance, security	2	*	*	*
Medical receptionists	7	*	*	*
Medical secretaries, transcribers	10	0.24%	0.39%	0.60%
Medical records	2	*	*	*
Other administrative support	6	*	*	*
Registered nurses	10	0.39%	0.62%	1.61%
Licensed practical nurses	2	*	*	*
Medical assistants, nurse aides	3	*	*	*
Clinical laboratory	0	*	*	*
Radiology and imaging	0	*	*	*
Other medical support services	1	0.02%	0.02%	0.02%
Total employed support staff cost	44	2.17%	3.62%	5.01%
Total employed support staff benefits	40	0.68%	0.97%	1.33%
Total contracted support staff	7	*	*	*
Total support staff cost	45	3.03%	4.54%	6.34%

Table 7d. FTE Staff per FTE Physician (Staff Categories)

	Anesthesiology			
	Count	25th %tile	Median	75th %tile
Administrative and Business Staff per FTE Physician	40	0.31	0.38	0.66
Front Office Staff per FTE Physician	17	0.06	0.10	0.19
Clinical Staff per FTE Physician	12	0.05	0.10	0.25
Ancillary Service Staff per FTE Physician	1	*	*	*

Table 7e. Staff Cost per FTE Physician (Staff Categories)

	Anesthesiology			
	Count	25th %tile	Median	75th %tile
Administrative and Business Staff Salary per FTE Physician	40	$ 11,274	$ 15,040	$ 23,964
Front Office Staff Salary per FTE Physician	17	$ 1,655	$ 2,266	$ 5,097
Clinical Staff Salary per FTE Physician	12	$ 2,175	$ 4,118	$ 9,903
Ancillary Service Staff Salary per FTE Physician	1	*	*	*

Table 7f. Staff Cost As a Percent of Total Medical Revenue (Staff Categories)

	Anesthesiology			
	Count	25th %tile	Median	75th %tile
Administrative and Business Staff Salary As % of Total Medical Revenue	40	2.33%	3.35%	4.05%
Front Office Staff Salary As % of Total Medical Revenue	17	0.29%	0.50%	0.81%
Clinical Staff Salary As % of Total Medical Revenue	12	0.40%	0.64%	1.85%
Ancillary Service Staff Salary As % of Total Medical Revenue	1	*	*	*

TABLE 8 ■ Cardiology, Not Hospital/Integrated Delivery System Owned

Table 8a. FTE Staff per FTE Physician

		Cardiology		
	Count	25th %tile	Median	75th %tile
General administrative	92	0.18	0.25	0.40
Business office	91	0.67	0.84	1.06
Managed care administrative	23	0.06	0.09	0.14
Information technology	39	0.07	0.12	0.15
Housekeeping, maintenance, security	8	*	*	*
Medical receptionists	92	0.48	0.66	0.99
Medical secretaries, transcribers	82	0.24	0.36	0.53
Medical records	88	0.25	0.36	0.54
Other administrative support	47	0.09	0.15	0.25
Registered nurses	88	0.42	0.67	1.13
Licensed practical nurses	54	0.11	0.22	0.34
Medical assistants, nurse aides	87	0.25	0.50	0.71
Clinical laboratory	22	0.09	0.16	0.25
Radiology and imaging	78	0.26	0.40	0.61
Other medical support services	58	0.23	0.35	0.74
Total employed support staff	95	3.74	4.99	6.10
Total contracted support staff	53	0.07	0.21	0.41
Total support staff	95	3.92	5.03	6.29

Table 8b. Staff Cost per FTE Physician

		Cardiology		
	Count	25th %tile	Median	75th %tile
General administrative	90	$ 13,196	$ 17,187	$ 26,510
Business office	89	$ 17,240	$ 21,976	$ 29,092
Managed care administrative	22	$ 2,140	$ 3,559	$ 6,546
Information technology	39	$ 2,618	$ 3,786	$ 5,475
Housekeeping, maintenance, security	8	*	*	*
Medical receptionists	90	$ 10,926	$ 15,366	$ 20,744
Medical secretaries, transcribers	82	$ 6,961	$ 9,763	$ 14,314
Medical records	86	$ 4,733	$ 7,128	$ 10,943
Other administrative support	45	$ 1,917	$ 4,482	$ 7,555
Registered nurses	86	$ 18,719	$ 27,453	$ 41,570
Licensed practical nurses	53	$ 3,247	$ 6,308	$ 11,817
Medical assistants, nurse aides	85	$ 6,562	$ 10,697	$ 16,794
Clinical laboratory	23	$ 2,779	$ 4,793	$ 7,080
Radiology and imaging	76	$ 10,832	$ 17,801	$ 25,642
Other medical support services	58	$ 7,558	$ 12,459	$ 26,475
Total employed support staff cost	94	$ 119,602	$ 156,101	$ 199,241
Total employed support staff benefits	92	$ 30,237	$ 37,281	$ 50,694
Total contracted support staff	57	$ 2,402	$ 6,110	$ 11,974
Total support staff cost	95	$ 157,476	$ 195,591	$ 250,994

TABLE 8 ■ Continued

Table 8c. Staff Cost As a Percent of Total Medical Revenue

	Cardiology			
	Count	25th %tile	Median	75th %tile
General administrative	90	1.54%	2.25%	2.84%
Business office	89	2.04%	2.65%	3.33%
Managed care administrative	22	0.25%	0.38%	0.77%
Information technology	39	0.31%	0.45%	0.63%
Housekeeping, maintenance, security	8	*	*	*
Medical receptionists	90	1.32%	1.79%	2.35%
Medical secretaries, transcribers	82	0.76%	1.06%	1.73%
Medical records	86	0.56%	0.86%	1.26%
Other administrative support	45	0.22%	0.46%	0.83%
Registered nurses	86	2.10%	3.55%	4.48%
Licensed practical nurses	53	0.38%	0.63%	1.23%
Medical assistants, nurse aides	85	0.71%	1.22%	2.10%
Clinical laboratory	23	0.28%	0.52%	0.82%
Radiology and imaging	76	1.19%	1.77%	2.69%
Other medical support services	58	0.83%	1.65%	2.64%
Total employed support staff cost	94	15.56%	17.78%	21.72%
Total employed support staff benefits	92	3.52%	4.58%	5.55%
Total contracted support staff	57	0.26%	0.81%	1.32%
Total support staff cost	95	19.37%	23.09%	27.88%

Table 8d. FTE Staff per FTE Physician (Staff Categories)

	Cardiology			
	Count	25th %tile	Median	75th %tile
Administrative and Business Staff per FTE Physician	93	0.97	1.20	1.57
Front Office Staff per FTE Physician	93	1.17	1.52	2.05
Clinical Staff per FTE Physician	92	0.97	1.33	1.77
Ancillary Service Staff per FTE Physician	88	0.47	0.73	1.00

Table 8e. Staff Cost per FTE Physician (Staff Categories)

	Cardiology			
	Count	25th %tile	Median	75th %tile
Administrative and Business Staff Salary per FTE Physician	91	$ 33,500	$ 42,580	$ 61,333
Front Office Staff Salary per FTE Physician	91	$ 28,055	$ 36,402	$ 46,165
Clinical Staff Salary per FTE Physician	90	$ 34,723	$ 44,326	$ 60,676
Ancillary Service Staff Salary per FTE Physician	86	$ 19,444	$ 27,571	$ 39,957

Table 8f. Staff Cost As a Percent of Total Medical Revenue (Staff Categories)

	Cardiology			
	Count	25th %tile	Median	75th %tile
Administrative and Business Staff Salary As % of Total Medical Revenue	91	4.08%	5.27%	6.36%
Front Office Staff Salary As % of Total Medical Revenue	91	3.23%	4.25%	5.02%
Clinical Staff Salary As % of Total Medical Revenue	90	4.13%	5.16%	6.61%
Ancillary Service Staff Salary As % of Total Medical Revenue	86	2.18%	2.76%	4.22%

TABLE 9 — Family Practice, Not Hospital/Integrated Delivery System Owned

Table 9a. FTE Staff per FTE Physician

Family Practice (Not Hospital / IDS Owned)

	Count	25th %tile	Median	75th %tile
General administrative	49	0.17	0.24	0.32
Business office	53	0.55	0.80	1.07
Managed care administrative	16	0.09	0.16	0.25
Information technology	6	*	*	*
Housekeeping, maintenance, security	13	0.08	0.14	0.33
Medical receptionists	51	0.68	1.00	1.25
Medical secretaries, transcribers	37	0.20	0.34	0.56
Medical records	40	0.27	0.43	0.65
Other administrative support	13	0.11	0.13	0.17
Registered nurses	41	0.23	0.44	0.77
Licensed practical nurses	46	0.25	0.40	0.79
Medical assistants, nurse aides	44	0.40	0.76	1.09
Clinical laboratory	36	0.24	0.34	0.51
Radiology and imaging	30	0.14	0.21	0.29
Other medical support services	8	*	*	*
Total employed support staff	56	4.00	4.60	5.29
Total contracted support staff	21	0.09	0.23	0.43
Total support staff	56	4.08	4.67	5.45

Table 9b. Staff Cost per FTE Physician

Family Practice (Not Hospital / IDS Owned)

	Count	25th %tile	Median	75th %tile
General administrative	48	$8,991	$12,635	$17,860
Business office	53	$13,324	$18,464	$24,872
Managed care administrative	16	$2,934	$3,806	$6,331
Information technology	6	*	*	*
Housekeeping, maintenance, security	13	$1,076	$3,284	$4,805
Medical receptionists	50	$12,591	$19,760	$22,529
Medical secretaries, transcribers	37	$3,609	$7,940	$11,442
Medical records	39	$4,134	$7,184	$11,954
Other administrative support	13	$1,621	$2,194	$4,150
Registered nurses	40	$7,162	$12,146	$24,512
Licensed practical nurses	44	$6,527	$10,102	$16,908
Medical assistants, nurse aides	43	$7,200	$15,044	$26,527
Clinical laboratory	35	$6,500	$9,692	$15,876
Radiology and imaging	29	$4,391	$7,043	$7,956
Other medical support services	9	*	*	*
Total employed support staff cost	56	$95,625	$111,325	$133,928
Total employed support staff benefits	52	$17,449	$25,379	$32,463
Total contracted support staff	22	$2,603	$4,131	$6,056
Total support staff cost	56	$118,138	$139,054	$168,937

TABLE 9 ■ Continued

Table 9c. Staff Cost As a Percent of Total Medical Revenue

Family Practice (Not Hospital / IDS Owned)

	Count	25th %tile	Median	75th %tile
General administrative	48	2.09%	2.51%	3.82%
Business office	53	3.16%	4.18%	5.06%
Managed care administrative	16	0.60%	0.87%	1.42%
Information technology	6	*	*	*
Housekeeping, maintenance, security	13	0.23%	0.56%	0.92%
Medical receptionists	50	3.06%	4.31%	5.43%
Medical secretaries, transcribers	37	1.04%	1.62%	2.28%
Medical records	39	1.13%	1.53%	2.40%
Other administrative support	13	0.35%	0.51%	1.16%
Registered nurses	40	1.62%	3.26%	4.73%
Licensed practical nurses	44	1.39%	2.37%	4.25%
Medical assistants, nurse aides	43	1.76%	3.72%	5.60%
Clinical laboratory	35	1.35%	2.34%	3.20%
Radiology and imaging	29	0.92%	1.20%	1.64%
Other medical support services	9	*	*	*
Total employed support staff cost	56	22.34%	25.59%	30.28%
Total employed support staff benefits	52	4.09%	5.72%	7.01%
Total contracted support staff	22	0.47%	0.83%	1.60%
Total support staff cost	56	27.67%	31.57%	36.71%

Table 9d. FTE Staff per FTE Physician (Staff Categories)

Family Practice (Not Hospital / IDS Owned)

	Count	25th %tile	Median	75th %tile
Administrative and Business Staff per FTE Physician	54	0.87	1.08	1.50
Front Office Staff per FTE Physician	52	1.42	1.62	2.00
Clinical Staff per FTE Physician	53	1.22	1.49	1.78
Ancillary Service Staff per FTE Physician	42	0.30	0.51	0.66

Table 9e. Staff Cost per FTE Physician (Staff Categories)

Family Practice (Not Hospital / IDS Owned)

	Count	25th %tile	Median	75th %tile
Administrative and Business Staff Salary per FTE Physician	53	$25,970	$31,852	$41,835
Front Office Staff Salary per FTE Physician	51	$22,497	$30,965	$38,636
Clinical Staff Salary per FTE Physician	52	$30,260	$35,759	$46,653
Ancillary Service Staff Salary per FTE Physician	42	$9,349	$13,401	$19,291

Table 9f. Staff Cost As a Percent of Total Medical Revenue (Staff Categories)

Family Practice (Not Hospital / IDS Owned)

	Count	25th %tile	Median	75th %tile
Administrative and Business Staff Salary As % of Total Medical Revenue	53	5.96%	7.13%	9.42%
Front Office Staff Salary As % of Total Medical Revenue	51	5.62%	6.68%	9.24%
Clinical Staff Salary As % of Total Medical Revenue	52	6.90%	8.59%	10.54%
Ancillary Service Staff Salary As % of Total Medical Revenue	42	2.05%	2.95%	4.81%

TABLE 10 — Family Practice, Hospital/Integrated Delivery System Owned

Table 10a. FTE Staff per FTE Physician

Family Practice (Hospital / IDS Owned)

	Count	25th %tile	Median	75th %tile
General administrative	15	0.10	0.18	0.32
Business office	32	0.32	0.50	1.61
Managed care administrative	7	0.05	0.14	0.21
Information technology	3	*	*	*
Housekeeping, maintenance, security	2	*	*	*
Medical receptionists	18	0.76	1.13	1.49
Medical secretaries, transcribers	20	0.22	0.33	0.43
Medical records	14	0.22	0.34	0.58
Other administrative support	16	0.16	1.08	2.00
Registered nurses	22	0.29	0.50	0.89
Licensed practical nurses	30	0.39	0.95	1.45
Medical assistants, nurse aides	24	0.23	0.45	0.82
Clinical laboratory	13	0.17	0.30	0.39
Radiology and imaging	11	0.14	0.20	0.33
Other medical support services	3	*	*	*
Total employed support staff	35	3.65	4.34	4.81
Total contracted support staff	7	*	*	*
Total support staff	40	3.79	4.47	5.28

Table 10b. Staff Cost per FTE Physician

Family Practice (Hospital / IDS Owned)

	Count	25th %tile	Median	75th %tile
General administrative	13	$5,746	$9,625	$12,661
Business office	30	$9,634	$18,005	$36,996
Managed care administrative	6	*	*	*
Information technology	2	*	*	*
Housekeeping, maintenance, security	1	*	*	*
Medical receptionists	16	$18,985	$23,705	$30,787
Medical secretaries, transcribers	18	$4,912	$8,665	$12,812
Medical records	12	$3,851	$5,665	$11,899
Other administrative support	14	$6,318	$32,799	$46,414
Registered nurses	20	$10,677	$15,329	$26,484
Licensed practical nurses	30	$11,094	$25,329	$35,943
Medical assistants, nurse aides	22	$5,135	$9,809	$18,680
Clinical laboratory	12	$5,987	$8,261	$9,713
Radiology and imaging	10	$4,168	$7,047	$10,304
Other medical support services	3	*	*	*
Total employed support staff cost	39	$89,629	$110,864	$126,765
Total employed support staff benefits	38	$17,807	$23,640	$28,357
Total contracted support staff	26	$4,185	$7,958	$12,999
Total support staff cost	40	$115,844	$138,863	$159,440

TABLE 10 ■ Continued

Table 10c. Staff Cost As a Percent of Total Medical Revenue

Family Practice (Hospital / IDS Owned)

	Count	25th %tile	Median	75th %tile
General administrative	13	1.33%	2.26%	3.25%
Business office	30	3.08%	4.40%	9.53%
Managed care administrative	6	*	*	*
Information technology	2	*	*	*
Housekeeping, maintenance, security	1	*	*	*
Medical receptionists	16	3.97%	6.61%	8.74%
Medical secretaries, transcribers	18	1.08%	1.78%	3.74%
Medical records	12	0.68%	1.70%	3.55%
Other administrative support	14	1.22%	6.75%	9.43%
Registered nurses	20	2.64%	4.34%	7.45%
Licensed practical nurses	30	3.12%	6.31%	8.24%
Medical assistants, nurse aides	22	0.94%	2.72%	4.16%
Clinical laboratory	12	1.15%	1.84%	2.12%
Radiology and imaging	10	0.75%	1.52%	2.00%
Other medical support services	3	*	*	*
Total employed support staff cost	39	22.58%	25.60%	30.00%
Total employed support staff benefits	38	4.73%	5.70%	6.41%
Total contracted support staff	26	0.76%	1.89%	3.00%
Total support staff cost	40	28.24%	32.78%	40.69%

Table 10d. FTE Staff per FTE Physician (Staff Categories)

Family Practice (Hospital / IDS Owned)

	Count	25th %tile	Median	75th %tile
Administrative and Business Staff per FTE Physician	34	0.39	0.55	1.79
Front Office Staff per FTE Physician	29	1.45	1.75	2.29
Clinical Staff per FTE Physician	35	1.29	1.60	1.98
Ancillary Service Staff per FTE Physician	20	0.18	0.32	0.42

Table 10e. Staff Cost per FTE Physician (Staff Categories)

Family Practice (Hospital / IDS Owned)

	Count	25th %tile	Median	75th %tile
Administrative and Business Staff Salary per FTE Physician	32	$ 14,870	$ 22,093	$ 39,130
Front Office Staff Salary per FTE Physician	27	$ 31,669	$ 39,814	$ 50,502
Clinical Staff Salary per FTE Physician	33	$ 34,359	$ 41,688	$ 56,811
Ancillary Service Staff Salary per FTE Physician	20	$ 4,396	$ 8,495	$ 10,333

Table 10f. Staff Cost As a Percent of Total Medical Revenue (Staff Categories)

Family Practice (Hospital / IDS Owned)

	Count	25th %tile	Median	75th %tile
Administrative and Business Staff Salary As % of Total Medical Revenue	32	3.40%	5.66%	10.24%
Front Office Staff Salary As % of Total Medical Revenue	27	8.03%	9.33%	12.78%
Clinical Staff Salary As % of Total Medical Revenue	33	8.17%	10.73%	13.59%
Ancillary Service Staff Salary As % of Total Medical Revenue	20	1.00%	1.94%	2.19%

TABLE 11 — Gastroenterology, Not Hospital/Integrated Delivery System Owned

Table 11a. FTE Staff per FTE Physician

		Gastroenterology		
	Count	25th %tile	Median	75th %tile
General administrative	21	0.16	0.25	0.40
Business office	21	0.52	0.75	1.03
Managed care administrative	1	*	*	*
Information technology	4	*	*	*
Housekeeping, maintenance, security	3	*	*	*
Medical receptionists	21	0.48	0.72	1.17
Medical secretaries, transcribers	16	0.16	0.28	0.50
Medical records	20	0.26	0.48	0.71
Other administrative support	6	*	*	*
Registered nurses	19	0.13	0.50	0.75
Licensed practical nurses	14	0.12	0.20	0.46
Medical assistants, nurse aides	19	0.31	0.53	1.00
Clinical laboratory	1	*	*	*
Radiology and imaging	2	*	*	*
Other medical support services	6	*	*	*
Total employed support staff	23	2.59	4.08	5.88
Total contracted support staff	10	0.16	0.25	0.38
Total support staff	23	2.84	4.08	6.57

Table 11b. Staff Cost per FTE Physician

		Gastroenterology		
	Count	25th %tile	Median	75th %tile
General administrative	20	$11,174	$16,239	$19,991
Business office	20	$14,396	$20,717	$27,037
Managed care administrative	1	*	*	*
Information technology	4	*	*	*
Housekeeping, maintenance, security	3	*	*	*
Medical receptionists	19	$10,633	$15,558	$24,031
Medical secretaries, transcribers	15	$3,710	$4,961	$11,166
Medical records	19	$4,427	$7,453	$14,951
Other administrative support	5	*	*	*
Registered nurses	17	$6,085	$23,043	$30,412
Licensed practical nurses	13	$3,395	$3,854	$13,377
Medical assistants, nurse aides	18	$8,053	$10,993	$21,639
Clinical laboratory	1	*	*	*
Radiology and imaging	2	*	*	*
Other medical support services	6	*	*	*
Total employed support staff cost	23	$73,650	$113,768	$172,636
Total employed support staff benefits	21	$22,257	$28,969	$35,304
Total contracted support staff	15	$1,273	$3,925	$7,149
Total support staff cost	23	$101,710	$146,514	$210,128

TABLE 11 ■ Continued

Table 11c. Staff Cost As a Percent of Total Medical Revenue

		Gastroenterology		
	Count	25th %tile	Median	75th %tile
General administrative	20	1.91%	2.39%	3.30%
Business office	20	2.61%	3.31%	4.22%
Managed care administrative	1	*	*	*
Information technology	4	*	*	*
Housekeeping, maintenance, security	3	*	*	*
Medical receptionists	19	1.85%	2.79%	4.11%
Medical secretaries, transcribers	15	0.62%	0.93%	1.38%
Medical records	19	0.83%	1.49%	2.23%
Other administrative support	5	*	*	*
Registered nurses	17	0.99%	3.35%	5.42%
Licensed practical nurses	13	0.56%	0.75%	2.24%
Medical assistants, nurse aides	18	1.28%	2.04%	3.26%
Clinical laboratory	1	*	*	*
Radiology and imaging	2	*	*	*
Other medical support services	6	*	*	*
Total employed support staff cost	23	12.48%	17.55%	22.51%
Total employed support staff benefits	21	3.76%	4.80%	5.68%
Total contracted support staff	15	0.17%	0.60%	1.14%
Total support staff cost	23	16.25%	22.72%	29.23%

Table 11d. FTE Staff per FTE Physician (Staff Categories)

		Gastroenterology		
	Count	25th %tile	Median	75th %tile
Administrative and Business Staff per FTE Physician	21	0.81	0.99	1.37
Front Office Staff per FTE Physician	21	0.95	1.53	2.61
Clinical Staff per FTE Physician	21	0.85	1.25	2.12
Ancillary Service Staff per FTE Physician	8	*	*	*

Table 11e. Staff Cost per FTE Physician (Staff Categories)

		Gastroenterology		
	Count	25th %tile	Median	75th %tile
Administrative and Business Staff Salary per FTE Physician	20	$ 29,023	$ 35,797	$ 48,660
Front Office Staff Salary per FTE Physician	19	$ 17,209	$ 26,197	$ 57,984
Clinical Staff Salary per FTE Physician	19	$ 23,462	$ 36,675	$ 54,376
Ancillary Service Staff Salary per FTE Physician	8	*	*	*

Table 11f. Staff Cost As a Percent of Total Medical Revenue (Staff Categories)

		Gastroenterology		
	Count	25th %tile	Median	75th %tile
Administrative and Business Staff Salary As % of Total Medical Revenue	20	4.90%	5.79%	7.31%
Front Office Staff Salary As % of Total Medical Revenue	19	3.32%	5.27%	7.45%
Clinical Staff Salary As % of Total Medical Revenue	19	3.69%	5.93%	7.83%
Ancillary Service Staff Salary As % of Total Medical Revenue	8	*	*	*

TABLE 12 — Hematology/Oncology, Not Hospital/Integrated Delivery System Owned

Table 12a. FTE Staff per FTE Physician

		Hematology / Oncology		
	Count	25th %tile	Median	75th %tile
General administrative	24	0.22	0.29	0.50
Business office	26	0.69	0.89	1.17
Managed care administrative	1	*	*	*
Information technology	5	*	*	*
Housekeeping, maintenance, security	4	*	*	*
Medical receptionists	26	0.56	0.82	1.08
Medical secretaries, transcribers	21	0.22	0.36	0.63
Medical records	21	0.25	0.40	0.52
Other administrative support	7	*	*	*
Registered nurses	25	0.92	1.33	1.58
Licensed practical nurses	12	0.13	0.33	0.56
Medical assistants, nurse aides	22	0.31	0.47	0.68
Clinical laboratory	20	0.39	0.50	0.76
Radiology and imaging	4	*	*	*
Other medical support services	9	*	*	*
Total employed support staff	26	4.16	4.89	7.19
Total contracted support staff	16	0.18	0.39	0.57
Total support staff	26	4.33	5.22	7.19

Table 12b. Staff Cost per FTE Physician

		Hematology / Oncology		
	Count	25th %tile	Median	75th %tile
General administrative	24	$ 15,575	$ 25,512	$ 32,018
Business office	26	$ 20,019	$ 29,415	$ 38,997
Managed care administrative	1	*	*	*
Information technology	5	*	*	*
Housekeeping, maintenance, security	4	*	*	*
Medical receptionists	26	$ 13,213	$ 18,861	$ 25,737
Medical secretaries, transcribers	21	$ 6,753	$ 10,084	$ 19,128
Medical records	21	$ 5,808	$ 7,635	$ 11,442
Other administrative support	7	*	*	*
Registered nurses	25	$ 44,817	$ 58,659	$ 74,409
Licensed practical nurses	12	$ 4,048	$ 9,679	$ 13,663
Medical assistants, nurse aides	23	$ 6,592	$ 11,451	$ 18,187
Clinical laboratory	20	$ 10,724	$ 15,442	$ 26,279
Radiology and imaging	4	*	*	*
Other medical support services	9	*	*	*
Total employed support staff cost	25	$ 144,080	$ 173,441	$ 249,254
Total employed support staff benefits	25	$ 28,040	$ 47,915	$ 64,757
Total contracted support staff	19	$ 2,375	$ 5,000	$ 13,758
Total support staff cost	26	$ 189,541	$ 231,587	$ 322,994

TABLE 12 ■ Continued

Table 12c. Staff Cost As a Percent of Total Medical Revenue

	Count	Hematology / Oncology 25th %tile	Median	75th %tile
General administrative	24	1.01%	1.41%	2.10%
Business office	26	1.27%	1.92%	2.38%
Managed care administrative	1	*	*	*
Information technology	5	*	*	*
Housekeeping, maintenance, security	4	*	*	*
Medical receptionists	26	0.70%	1.17%	1.79%
Medical secretaries, transcribers	21	0.44%	0.68%	0.98%
Medical records	21	0.29%	0.51%	0.76%
Other administrative support	7	*	*	*
Registered nurses	25	2.76%	3.29%	4.30%
Licensed practical nurses	12	0.37%	0.51%	0.89%
Medical assistants, nurse aides	23	0.35%	0.82%	1.21%
Clinical laboratory	20	0.71%	1.00%	1.48%
Radiology and imaging	4	*	*	*
Other medical support services	9	*	*	*
Total employed support staff cost	25	9.30%	11.36%	13.80%
Total employed support staff benefits	25	2.01%	2.69%	3.52%
Total contracted support staff	19	0.14%	0.28%	0.83%
Total support staff cost	26	13.08%	14.98%	16.78%

Table 12d. FTE Staff per FTE Physician (Staff Categories)

	Count	Hematology / Oncology 25th %tile	Median	75th %tile
Administrative and Business Staff per FTE Physician	26	0.93	1.23	1.75
Front Office Staff per FTE Physician	26	1.08	1.63	1.93
Clinical Staff per FTE Physician	25	1.40	1.90	2.29
Ancillary Service Staff per FTE Physician	22	0.30	0.52	0.96

Table 12e. Staff Cost per FTE Physician (Staff Categories)

	Count	Hematology / Oncology 25th %tile	Median	75th %tile
Administrative and Business Staff Salary per FTE Physician	26	$ 35,292	$ 57,003	$ 75,311
Front Office Staff Salary per FTE Physician	26	$ 27,307	$ 39,611	$ 49,640
Clinical Staff Salary per FTE Physician	25	$ 56,677	$ 77,040	$ 93,119
Ancillary Service Staff Salary per FTE Physician	22	$ 9,892	$ 19,396	$ 36,989

Table 12f. Staff Cost As a Percent of Total Medical Revenue (Staff Categories)

	Count	Hematology / Oncology 25th %tile	Median	75th %tile
Administrative and Business Staff Salary As % of Total Medical Revenue	26	2.32%	3.29%	4.29%
Front Office Staff Salary As % of Total Medical Revenue	26	1.79%	2.49%	2.95%
Clinical Staff Salary As % of Total Medical Revenue	25	3.95%	4.46%	5.64%
Ancillary Service Staff Salary As % of Total Medical Revenue	22	0.68%	1.20%	2.08%

TABLE 13 — Internal Medicine, Not Hospital/Integrated Delivery System Owned

Table 13a. FTE Staff per FTE Physician

Internal Medicine (Not Hospital / IDS Owned)

	Count	25th %tile	Median	75th %tile
General administrative	17	0.16	0.20	0.48
Business office	17	0.34	0.54	0.75
Managed care administrative	5	*	*	*
Information technology	4	*	*	*
Housekeeping, maintenance, security	3	*	*	*
Medical receptionists	15	0.30	0.67	1.28
Medical secretaries, transcribers	10	0.20	0.27	0.54
Medical records	14	0.24	0.36	0.56
Other administrative support	4	*	*	*
Registered nurses	12	0.23	0.62	0.98
Licensed practical nurses	12	0.33	0.41	0.64
Medical assistants, nurse aides	15	0.33	0.60	1.11
Clinical laboratory	9	*	*	*
Radiology and imaging	7	*	*	*
Other medical support services	4	*	*	*
Total employed support staff	19	3.01	4.30	6.05
Total contracted support staff	11	0.11	0.20	0.29
Total support staff	19	3.01	4.30	6.07

Table 13b. Staff Cost per FTE Physician

Internal Medicine (Not Hospital / IDS Owned)

	Count	25th %tile	Median	75th %tile
General administrative	18	$ 8,123	$ 10,342	$ 18,936
Business office	18	$ 9,803	$ 12,956	$ 21,924
Managed care administrative	5	*	*	*
Information technology	4	*	*	*
Housekeeping, maintenance, security	3	*	*	*
Medical receptionists	16	$ 9,609	$ 15,347	$ 27,294
Medical secretaries, transcribers	11	$ 6,160	$ 7,800	$ 11,649
Medical records	14	$ 3,373	$ 6,541	$ 9,622
Other administrative support	6	*	*	*
Registered nurses	13	$ 10,511	$ 21,002	$ 33,779
Licensed practical nurses	13	$ 7,539	$ 9,362	$ 15,831
Medical assistants, nurse aides	16	$ 6,093	$ 11,893	$ 26,690
Clinical laboratory	10	$ 6,045	$ 11,305	$ 18,248
Radiology and imaging	8	*	*	*
Other medical support services	5	*	*	*
Total employed support staff cost	19	$ 81,781	$ 122,430	$ 152,951
Total employed support staff benefits	18	$ 18,631	$ 27,746	$ 35,657
Total contracted support staff	15	$ 2,737	$ 4,732	$ 10,951
Total support staff cost	19	$ 105,966	$ 148,974	$ 205,371

TABLE 13 ■ Continued

Table 13c. Staff Cost As a Percent of Total Medical Revenue

	\multicolumn{4}{l}{Internal Medicine (Not Hospital / IDS Owned)}
	Count	25th %tile	Median	75th %tile
General administrative	18	1.74%	2.26%	3.86%
Business office	18	2.02%	3.15%	4.27%
Managed care administrative	5	*	*	*
Information technology	4	*	*	*
Housekeeping, maintenance, security	3	*	*	*
Medical receptionists	16	1.94%	3.10%	5.30%
Medical secretaries, transcribers	11	0.94%	1.60%	2.61%
Medical records	14	0.80%	1.62%	1.92%
Other administrative support	6	*	*	*
Registered nurses	13	3.19%	4.41%	7.81%
Licensed practical nurses	13	1.55%	2.39%	3.60%
Medical assistants, nurse aides	16	1.39%	2.84%	5.32%
Clinical laboratory	10	1.15%	2.00%	4.23%
Radiology and imaging	8	*	*	*
Other medical support services	5	*	*	*
Total employed support staff cost	19	21.53%	24.10%	27.54%
Total employed support staff benefits	8	4.55%	5.46%	6.66%
Total contracted support staff	15	0.60%	0.85%	2.03%
Total support staff cost	19	25.54%	30.30%	34.54%

Table 13d. FTE Staff per FTE Physician (Staff Categories)

	\multicolumn{4}{l}{Internal Medicine (Not Hospital / IDS Owned)}
	Count	25th %tile	Median	75th %tile
Administrative and Business Staff per FTE Physician	17	0.65	0.89	1.41
Front Office Staff per FTE Physician	17	0.86	1.35	1.71
Clinical Staff per FTE Physician	16	1.03	1.41	2.09
Ancillary Service Staff per FTE Physician	11	0.20	0.51	0.85

Table 13e. Staff Cost As a Percent of Total Medical Revenue (Staff Categories)

	\multicolumn{4}{l}{Internal Medicine (Not Hospital / IDS Owned)}
	Count	25th %tile	Median	75th %tile
Administrative and Business Staff Salary per FTE Physician	18	$ 22,369	$ 27,915	$ 47,410
Front Office Staff Salary per FTE Physician	18	$ 18,209	$ 24,782	$ 42,427
Clinical Staff Salary per FTE Physician	17	$ 31,065	$ 39,892	$ 48,727
Ancillary Service Staff Salary per FTE Physician	12	$ 6,249	$ 19,674	$ 34,151

Table 13f. Staff Cost per FTE Physician (Staff Categories)

	\multicolumn{4}{l}{Internal Medicine (Not Hospital / IDS Owned)}
	Count	25th %tile	Median	75th %tile
Administrative and Business Staff Salary As % of Total Medical Revenue	18	4.70%	6.29%	8.69%
Front Office Staff Salary As % of Total Medical Revenue	18	4.50%	5.35%	6.90%
Clinical Staff Salary As % of Total Medical Revenue	17	7.20%	7.83%	10.74%
Ancillary Service Staff Salary As % of Total Medical Revenue	12	1.50%	3.71%	5.25%

TABLE 14 — Internal Medicine, Hospital/Integrated Delivery System Owned

Table 14a. FTE Staff per FTE Physician

Internal Medicine (Hospital / IDS Owned)

	Count	25th %tile	Median	75th %tile
General administrative	14	0.13	0.22	0.30
Business office	17	0.36	0.67	1.05
Managed care administrative	2	*	*	*
Information technology	1	*	*	*
Housekeeping, maintenance, security	2	*	*	*
Medical receptionists	12	0.54	0.82	1.33
Medical secretaries, transcribers	7	*	*	*
Medical records	14	0.31	0.44	0.60
Other administrative support	10	0.12	0.22	0.38
Registered nurses	18	0.33	0.50	0.73
Licensed practical nurses	18	0.33	0.48	0.71
Medical assistants, nurse aides	16	0.13	0.32	0.63
Clinical laboratory	11	0.18	0.28	0.33
Radiology and imaging	6	*	*	*
Other medical support services	5	*	*	*
Total employed support staff	18	3.18	4.09	4.84
Total contracted support staff	10	0.03	0.28	0.74
Total support staff	21	2.93	3.81	5.01

Table 14b. Staff Cost per FTE Physician

Internal Medicine (Hospital / IDS Owned)

	Count	25th %tile	Median	75th %tile
General administrative	10	$8,304	$12,467	$17,017
Business office	13	$9,312	$22,117	$32,791
Managed care administrative	1	*	*	*
Information technology	0	*	*	*
Housekeeping, maintenance, security	1	*	*	*
Medical receptionists	8	*	*	*
Medical secretaries, transcribers	6	*	*	*
Medical records	10	$6,336	$8,378	$13,843
Other administrative support	9	*	*	*
Registered nurses	14	$6,311	$17,068	$25,558
Licensed practical nurses	14	$8,253	$13,461	$18,967
Medical assistants, nurse aides	12	$4,006	$8,030	$12,334
Clinical laboratory	8	*	*	*
Radiology and imaging	6	*	*	*
Other medical support services	4	*	*	*
Total employed support staff cost	19	$84,594	$94,883	$133,476
Total employed support staff benefits	19	$15,623	$21,558	$26,340
Total contracted support staff	16	$704	$9,423	$14,353
Total support staff cost	21	$102,894	$114,190	$172,494

TABLE 14 ■ Continued

Table 14c. Staff Cost As a Percent of Total Medical Revenue

Internal Medicine (Hospital / IDS Owned)

	Count	25th %tile	Median	75th %tile
General administrative	10	2.08%	2.82%	4.48%
Business office	13	2.75%	5.34%	8.02%
Managed care administrative	1	*	*	*
Information technology	0	*	*	*
Housekeeping, maintenance, security	1	*	*	*
Medical receptionists	8	*	*	*
Medical secretaries, transcribers	6	*	*	*
Medical records	10	1.34%	2.57%	3.26%
Other administrative support	9	*	*	*
Registered nurses	14	2.05%	3.68%	6.01%
Licensed practical nurses	14	2.13%	3.55%	5.03%
Medical assistants, nurse aides	12	1.03%	1.98%	4.19%
Clinical laboratory	8	*	*	*
Radiology and imaging	6	*	*	*
Other medical support services	4	*	*	*
Total employed support staff cost	19	25.14%	30.94%	34.76%
Total employed support staff benefits	19	4.80%	5.79%	6.87%
Total contracted support staff	16	0.16%	1.95%	5.59%
Total support staff cost	21	32.55%	36.70%	44.27%

Table 14d. FTE Staff per FTE Physician (Staff Categories)

Internal Medicine (Hospital / IDS Owned)

	Count	25th %tile	Median	75th %tile
Administrative and Business Staff per FTE Physician	17	0.67	1.00	1.20
Front Office Staff per FTE Physician	17	0.84	1.08	2.05
Clinical Staff per FTE Physician	18	1.05	1.33	1.75
Ancillary Service Staff per FTE Physician	13	0.30	0.38	0.70

Table 14e. Staff Cost per FTE Physician (Staff Categories)

Internal Medicine (Hospital / IDS Owned)

	Count	25th %tile	Median	75th %tile
Administrative and Business Staff Salary per FTE Physician	13	$ 20,683	$ 30,340	$ 47,494
Front Office Staff Salary per FTE Physician	13	$ 19,912	$ 29,076	$ 43,434
Clinical Staff Salary per FTE Physician	14	$ 31,706	$ 36,289	$ 45,752
Ancillary Service Staff Salary per FTE Physician	9	*	*	*

Table 14f. Staff Cost As a Percent of Total Medical Revenue (Staff Categories)

Internal Medicine (Hospital / IDS Owned)

	Count	25th %tile	Median	75th %tile
Administrative and Business Staff Salary As % of Total Medical Revenue	13	4.77%	8.30%	11.10%
Front Office Staff Salary As % of Total Medical Revenue	13	4.74%	9.10%	12.08%
Clinical Staff Salary As % of Total Medical Revenue	14	7.55%	9.83%	12.22%
Ancillary Service Staff Salary As % of Total Medical Revenue	9	*	*	*

TABLE 15 — Neurology, Not Hospital/Integrated Delivery System Owned

Table 15a. FTE Staff per FTE Physician

		Neurology		
	Count	25th %tile	Median	75th %tile
General administrative	9	*	*	*
Business office	10	0.63	0.73	1.33
Managed care administrative	1	*	*	*
Information technology	1	*	*	*
Housekeeping, maintenance, security	1	*	*	*
Medical receptionists	10	0.29	0.54	1.50
Medical secretaries, transcribers	9	*	*	*
Medical records	8	*	*	*
Other administrative support	0	*	*	*
Registered nurses	4	*	*	*
Licensed practical nurses	2	*	*	*
Medical assistants, nurse aides	5	*	*	*
Clinical laboratory	4	*	*	*
Radiology and imaging	4	*	*	*
Other medical support services	7	*	*	*
Total employed support staff	10	3.53	4.09	4.87
Total contracted support staff	7	*	*	*
Total support staff	10	3.74	4.33	5.19

Table 15b. Staff Cost per FTE Physician

		Neurology		
	Count	25th %tile	Median	75th %tile
General administrative	9	*	*	*
Business office	10	$ 15,094	$ 22,314	$ 34,387
Managed care administrative	1	*	*	*
Information technology	1	*	*	*
Housekeeping, maintenance, security	1	*	*	*
Medical receptionists	10	$ 5,311	$ 12,124	$ 37,897
Medical secretaries, transcribers	9	*	*	*
Medical records	8	*	*	*
Other administrative support	0	*	*	*
Registered nurses	4	*	*	*
Licensed practical nurses	2	*	*	*
Medical assistants, nurse aides	5	*	*	*
Clinical laboratory	4	*	*	*
Radiology and imaging	4	*	*	*
Other medical support services	7	*	*	*
Total employed support staff cost	10	$ 94,968	$ 128,359	$ 150,621
Total employed support staff benefits	8	*	*	*
Total contracted support staff	7	*	*	*
Total support staff cost	10	$ 115,662	$ 149,828	$ 205,764

TABLE 15 ■ Continued

Table 15c. Staff Cost As a Percent of Total Medical Revenue

		Neurology		
	Count	25th %tile	Median	75th %tile
General administrative	9	*	*	*
Business office	10	2.72%	3.66%	6.00%
Managed care administrative	1	*	*	*
Information technology	1	*	*	*
Housekeeping, maintenance, security	1	*	*	*
Medical receptionists	10	1.41%	2.55%	6.23%
Medical secretaries, transcribers	9	*	*	*
Medical records	8	*	*	*
Other administrative support	0	*	*	*
Registered nurses	4	*	*	*
Licensed practical nurses	2	*	*	*
Medical assistants, nurse aides	5	*	*	*
Clinical laboratory	4	*	*	*
Radiology and imaging	4	*	*	*
Other medical support services	7	*	*	*
Total employed support staff cost	10	20.10%	24.69%	28.02%
Total employed support staff benefits	8	*	*	*
Total contracted support staff	7	*	*	*
Total support staff cost	10	25.56%	31.74%	35.88%

Table 15d. FTE Staff per FTE Physician (Staff Categories)

		Neurology		
	Count	25th %tile	Median	75th %tile
Administrative and Business Staff per FTE Physician	10	0.76	1.06	1.74
Front Office Staff per FTE Physician	10	1.06	1.56	2.29
Clinical Staff per FTE Physician	7	*	*	*
Ancillary Service Staff per FTE Physician	10	0.42	0.76	1.67

Table 15e. Staff Cost per FTE physician (Staff Categories)

		Neurology		
	Count	25th %tile	Median	75th %tile
Administrative and Business Staff Salary per FTE Physician	10	$ 27,136	$ 38,690	$ 59,655
Front Office Staff Salary per FTE Physician	10	$ 24,184	$ 36,037	$ 53,254
Clinical Staff Salary per FTE Physician	7	*	*	*
Ancillary Service Staff Salary per FTE Physician	10	$ 11,095	$ 29,520	$ 55,139

Table 15f. Staff Cost As a Percent of Total Medical Revenue (Staff Categories)

		Neurology		
	Count	25th %tile	Median	75th %tile
Administrative and Business Staff Salary As % of Total Medical Revenue	10	5.49%	6.33%	8.10%
Front Office Staff Salary As % of Total Medical Revenue	10	5.02%	8.12%	11.47%
Clinical Staff Salary As % of Total Medical Revenue	7	*	*	*
Ancillary Service Staff Salary As % of Total Medical Revenue	10	2.24%	6.09%	7.95%

TABLE 16 — Obstetrics/Gynecology, Not Hospital/Integrated Delivery System Owned

Table 16a. FTE Staff per FTE Physician

	Count	Obstetrics / Gynecology 25th %tile	Median	75th %tile
General administrative	46	0.17	0.21	0.33
Business office	48	0.51	0.67	0.92
Managed care administrative	5	*	*	*
Information technology	5	*	*	*
Housekeeping, maintenance, security	3	*	*	*
Medical receptionists	48	0.76	0.98	1.12
Medical secretaries, transcribers	28	0.14	0.20	0.33
Medical records	43	0.21	0.33	0.50
Other administrative support	18	0.20	0.41	0.65
Registered nurses	40	0.38	0.55	0.99
Licensed practical nurses	36	0.22	0.35	0.60
Medical assistants, nurse aides	43	0.47	1.00	1.43
Clinical laboratory	20	0.16	0.29	0.38
Radiology and imaging	31	0.16	0.20	0.29
Other medical support services	8	*	*	*
Total employed support staff	49	3.70	4.65	5.75
Total contracted support staff	25	0.06	0.15	0.21
Total support staff	50	3.87	4.69	5.84

Table 16b. Staff Cost per FTE Physician

	Count	Obstetrics / Gynecology 25th %tile	Median	75th %tile
General administrative	46	$ 10,122	$ 14,329	$ 18,705
Business office	47	$ 14,705	$ 18,560	$ 23,830
Managed care administrative	6	*	*	*
Information technology	6	*	*	*
Housekeeping, maintenance, security	3	*	*	*
Medical receptionists	47	$ 14,928	$ 20,866	$ 25,750
Medical secretaries, transcribers	27	$ 3,180	$ 4,671	$ 8,013
Medical records	42	$ 3,450	$ 7,113	$ 10,839
Other administrative support	18	$ 4,470	$ 7,785	$ 14,531
Registered nurses	39	$ 9,167	$ 18,346	$ 36,522
Licensed practical nurses	35	$ 7,536	$ 10,561	$ 16,555
Medical assistants, nurse aides	42	$ 13,664	$ 22,660	$ 32,639
Clinical laboratory	20	$ 3,253	$ 7,435	$ 12,699
Radiology and imaging	30	$ 6,260	$ 9,216	$ 12,917
Other medical support services	10	$ 1,475	$ 2,938	$ 5,497
Total employed support staff cost	50	$ 102,487	$ 121,262	$ 155,350
Total employed support staff benefits	49	$ 24,381	$ 30,205	$ 37,384
Total contracted support staff	28	$ 916	$ 2,892	$ 6,655
Total support staff cost	50	$ 132,147	$ 149,448	$ 190,193

TABLE 16 ■ Continued

Table 16c. Staff Cost As a Percent of Total Medical Revenue

	Count	Obstetrics / Gynecology 25th %tile	Median	75th %tile
General administrative	46	1.84%	2.52%	2.89%
Business office	47	2.41%	3.23%	3.89%
Managed care administrative	6	*	*	*
Information technology	6	*	*	*
Housekeeping, maintenance, security	3	*	*	*
Medical receptionists	47	2.65%	3.31%	4.29%
Medical secretaries, transcribers	27	0.53%	0.74%	1.59%
Medical records	42	0.73%	1.20%	1.59%
Other administrative support	18	0.79%	1.04%	1.92%
Registered nurses	39	1.81%	3.21%	5.23%
Licensed practical nurses	35	1.08%	1.77%	2.86%
Medical assistants, nurse aides	42	2.16%	3.65%	4.69%
Clinical laboratory	20	0.57%	1.16%	1.95%
Radiology and imaging	30	1.01%	1.55%	2.11%
Other medical support services	10	0.22%	0.37%	0.93%
Total employed support staff cost	50	19.69%	21.10%	22.07%
Total employed support staff benefits	49	4.14%	5.03%	6.06%
Total contracted support staff	28	0.21%	0.60%	1.13%
Total support staff cost	50	24.35%	25.86%	27.85%

Table 16d. FTE Staff per FTE Physician (Staff Categories)

	Count	Obstetrics / Gynecology 25th %tile	Median	75th %tile
Administrative and Business Staff per FTE Physician	48	0.73	0.95	1.21
Front Office Staff per FTE Physician	48	1.22	1.55	1.98
Clinical Staff per FTE Physician	49	1.38	1.71	2.29
Ancillary Service Staff per FTE Physician	37	0.20	0.30	0.47

Table 16e. Staff Cost per FTE Physician (Staff Categories)

	Count	Obstetrics / Gynecology 25th %tile	Median	75th %tile
Administrative and Business Staff Salary per FTE Physician	47	$ 26,590	$ 32,315	$ 42,106
Front Office Staff Salary per FTE Physician	47	$ 26,690	$ 33,726	$ 40,706
Clinical Staff Salary per FTE Physician	48	$ 33,129	$ 44,817	$ 63,826
Ancillary Service Staff Salary per FTE Physician	36	$ 8,140	$ 11,741	$ 22,210

Table 16f. Staff Cost As a Percent of Total Medical Revenue (Staff Categories)

	Count	Obstetrics / Gynecology 25th %tile	Median	75th %tile
Administrative and Business Staff Salary As % of Total Medical Revenue	47	4.69%	5.87%	6.98%
Front Office Staff Salary As % of Total Medical Revenue	47	4.37%	5.28%	6.62%
Clinical Staff Salary As % of Total Medical Revenue	48	6.44%	7.53%	8.88%
Ancillary Service Staff Salary As % of Total Medical Revenue	36	1.34%	1.85%	2.80%

TABLE 17 — Obstetrics/Gynecology, Hospital/Integrated Delivery System Owned

Table 17a. FTE Staff per FTE Physician

Obstetrics / Gynecology (Hospital / IDS Owned)

	Count	25th %tile	Median	75th %tile
General administrative	16	0.12	0.26	0.32
Business office	18	0.64	1.34	2.08
Managed care administrative	1	*	*	*
Information technology	8	*	*	*
Housekeeping, maintenance, security	2	*	*	*
Medical receptionists	13	0.01	0.15	0.66
Medical secretaries, transcribers	9	*	*	*
Medical records	8	*	*	*
Other administrative support	8	*	*	*
Registered nurses	16	0.22	0.48	0.88
Licensed practical nurses	18	0.18	0.35	0.74
Medical assistants, nurse aides	18	0.25	0.49	0.95
Clinical laboratory	5	*	*	*
Radiology and imaging	8	*	*	*
Other medical support services	6	*	*	*
Total employed support staff	21	3.18	3.72	4.99
Total contracted support staff	12	0.08	0.29	0.58
Total support staff	22	3.40	3.82	5.12

Table 17b. Staff Cost per FTE Physician

Obstetrics / Gynecology (Hospital / IDS Owned)

	Count	25th %tile	Median	75th %tile
General administrative	15	$ 5,923	$ 11,609	$ 17,591
Business office	17	$ 19,011	$ 35,711	$ 52,146
Managed care administrative	0	*	*	*
Information technology	7	*	*	*
Housekeeping, maintenance, security	1	*	*	*
Medical receptionists	12	$ 240	$ 1,547	$ 14,624
Medical secretaries, transcribers	8	*	*	*
Medical records	7	*	*	*
Other administrative support	7	*	*	*
Registered nurses	15	$ 8,039	$ 18,408	$ 31,149
Licensed practical nurses	17	$ 4,058	$ 8,269	$ 20,160
Medical assistants, nurse aides	17	$ 6,532	$ 12,238	$ 21,019
Clinical laboratory	5	*	*	*
Radiology and imaging	8	*	*	*
Other medical support services	5	*	*	*
Total employed support staff cost	21	$ 73,564	$ 101,279	$ 133,257
Total employed support staff benefits	21	$ 4,888	$ 15,283	$ 19,728
Total contracted support staff	10	$ 2,061	$ 4,069	$ 12,528
Total support staff cost	22	$ 86,285	$ 121,904	$ 147,186

TABLE 17 Continued

Table 17c. Staff Cost As a Percent of Total Medical Revenue

Obstetrics / Gynecology (Hospital / IDS Owned)

	Count	25th %tile	Median	75th %tile
General administrative	15	1.90%	2.62%	3.47%
Business office	17	4.24%	7.39%	11.95%
Managed care administrative	0	*	*	*
Information technology	7	*	*	*
Housekeeping, maintenance, security	1	*	*	*
Medical receptionists	12	0.10%	0.35%	2.76%
Medical secretaries, transcribers	8	*	*	*
Medical records	7	*	*	*
Other administrative support	7	*	*	*
Registered nurses	15	1.79%	3.99%	7.19%
Licensed practical nurses	17	1.48%	2.22%	4.29%
Medical assistants, nurse aides	17	1.27%	2.73%	4.97%
Clinical laboratory	5	*	*	*
Radiology and imaging	8	*	*	*
Other medical support services	5	*	*	*
Total employed support staff cost	21	17.09%	22.68%	30.07%
Total employed support staff benefits	21	1.78%	2.97%	4.77%
Total contracted support staff	10	0.42%	0.58%	1.78%
Total support staff cost	22	20.75%	27.46%	31.89%

Table 17d. FTE Staff per FTE Physician (Staff Categories)

Obstetrics / Gynecology (Hospital / IDS Owned)

	Count	25th %tile	Median	75th %tile
Administrative and Business Staff per FTE Physician	19	0.97	1.60	2.38
Front Office Staff per FTE Physician	18	0.29	0.76	1.23
Clinical Staff per FTE Physician	20	0.98	1.46	1.75
Ancillary Service Staff per FTE Physician	12	0.23	0.36	0.63

Table 17e. Staff Cost per FTE Physician (Staff Categories)

Obstetrics / Gynecology (Hospital / IDS Owned)

	Count	25th %tile	Median	75th %tile
Administrative and Business Staff Salary per FTE Physician	18	$ 30,767	$ 41,814	$ 65,106
Front Office Staff Salary per FTE Physician	17	$ 6,675	$ 11,787	$ 26,354
Clinical Staff Salary per FTE Physician	19	$ 29,080	$ 38,151	$ 54,302
Ancillary Service Staff Salary per FTE Physician	11	$ 7,219	$ 13,877	$ 17,679

Table 17f. Staff Cost As a Percent of Total Medical Revenue (Staff Categories)

Obstetrics / Gynecology (Hospital / IDS Owned)

	Count	25th %tile	Median	75th %tile
Administrative and Business Staff Salary As % of Total Medical Revenue	18	6.00%	10.07%	14.30%
Front Office Staff Salary As % of Total Medical Revenue	17	1.19%	3.38%	5.07%
Clinical Staff Salary As % of Total Medical Revenue	19	6.57%	8.66%	12.23%
Ancillary Service Staff Salary As % of Total Medical Revenue	11	1.58%	2.29%	2.89%

TABLE 18 — Ophthalmology, Not Hospital/Integrated Delivery System Owned

Table 18a. FTE Staff per FTE Physician

		Ophthalmology		
	Count	25th %tile	Median	75th %tile
General administrative	21	0.26	0.40	0.54
Business office	21	0.71	0.97	1.24
Managed care administrative	1	*	*	*
Information technology	5	*	*	*
Housekeeping, maintenance, security	6	*	*	*
Medical receptionists	21	1.29	1.56	2.17
Medical secretaries, transcribers	14	0.17	0.22	0.38
Medical records	16	0.22	0.30	0.48
Other administrative support	9	*	*	*
Registered nurses	9	*	*	*
Licensed practical nurses	4	*	*	*
Medical assistants, nurse aides	18	1.85	2.71	3.44
Clinical laboratory	3	*	*	*
Radiology and imaging	0	*	*	*
Other medical support services	17	0.56	1.33	2.28
Total employed support staff	20	6.34	7.35	9.28
Total contracted support staff	4	*	*	*
Total support staff	21	6.35	7.58	10.07

Table 18b. Staff Cost per FTE Physician

		Ophthalmology		
	Count	25th %tile	Median	75th %tile
General administrative	21	$ 18,155	$ 21,684	$ 32,409
Business office	21	$ 14,233	$ 25,699	$ 31,665
Managed care administrative	1	*	*	*
Information technology	5	*	*	*
Housekeeping, maintenance, security	6	*	*	*
Medical receptionists	21	$ 23,260	$ 35,520	$ 44,650
Medical secretaries, transcribers	14	$ 4,111	$ 5,867	$ 11,136
Medical records	16	$ 3,441	$ 4,797	$ 9,865
Other administrative support	9	*	*	*
Registered nurses	9	*	*	*
Licensed practical nurses	4	*	*	*
Medical assistants, nurse aides	18	$ 54,139	$ 68,804	$ 98,512
Clinical laboratory	3	*	*	*
Radiology and imaging	0	*	*	*
Other medical support services	17	$ 18,790	$ 39,373	$ 56,505
Total employed support staff cost	21	$ 170,068	$ 202,117	$ 247,992
Total employed support staff benefits	21	$ 37,775	$ 52,513	$ 71,383
Total contracted support staff	6	*	*	*
Total support staff cost	21	$ 216,162	$ 261,429	$ 325,219

TABLE 18 ■ Continued

Table 18c. Staff Cost As a Percent of Total Medical Revenue

		Ophthalmology		
	Count	25th %tile	Median	75th %tile
General administrative	21	1.97%	2.66%	3.68%
Business office	21	1.84%	2.57%	3.72%
Managed care administrative	1	*	*	*
Information technology	5	*	*	*
Housekeeping, maintenance, security	6	*	*	*
Medical receptionists	21	2.74%	4.00%	4.40%
Medical secretaries, transcribers	14	0.42%	0.66%	1.01%
Medical records	16	0.37%	0.60%	1.05%
Other administrative support	9	*	*	*
Registered nurses	9	*	*	*
Licensed practical nurses	4	*	*	*
Medical assistants, nurse aides	18	6.94%	8.74%	10.21%
Clinical laboratory	3	*	*	*
Radiology and imaging	0	*	*	*
Other medical support services	17	2.42%	4.38%	5.89%
Total employed support staff cost	21	21.00%	22.86%	26.38%
Total employed support staff benefits	21	4.80%	6.48%	7.28%
Total contracted support staff	6	*	*	*
Total support staff cost	21	26.34%	29.34%	33.98%

Table 18d. FTE Staff per FTE Physician (Staff Categories)

		Ophthalmology		
	Count	25th %tile	Median	75th %tile
Administrative and Business Staff per FTE Physician	21	1.19	1.61	1.80
Front Office Staff per FTE Physician	21	1.54	2.25	2.83
Clinical Staff per FTE Physician	20	2.30	2.88	3.79
Ancillary Service Staff per FTE Physician	17	0.62	1.35	3.04

Table 18e. Staff Cost per FTE physician (Staff Categories)

		Ophthalmology		
	Count	25th %tile	Median	75th %tile
Administrative and Business Staff Salary per FTE Physician	21	$ 42,485	$ 52,652	$ 60,546
Front Office Staff Salary per FTE Physician	21	$ 30,475	$ 47,553	$ 61,490
Clinical Staff Salary per FTE Physician	20	$ 69,750	$ 79,472	$ 98,189
Ancillary Service Staff Salary per FTE Physician	17	$ 21,465	$ 43,534	$ 76,013

Table 18f. Staff Cost As a Percent of Total Medical Revenue (Staff Categories)

		Ophthalmology		
	Count	25th %tile	Median	75th %tile
Administrative and Business Staff Salary As % of Total Medical Revenue	21	4.43%	5.28%	6.91%
Front Office Staff Salary As % of Total Medical Revenue	21	4.10%	5.00%	6.37%
Clinical Staff Salary As % of Total Medical Revenue	20	7.22%	9.45%	10.52%
Ancillary Service Staff Salary As % of Total Medical Revenue	17	2.42%	5.48%	8.69%

TABLE 19 ■ Orthopedic Surgery, Not Hospital/Integrated Delivery System Owned

Table 19a. FTE Staff per FTE Physician

		Orthopedic Surgery		
	Count	25th %tile	Median	75th %tile
General administrative	116	0.17	0.25	0.35
Business office	118	0.67	0.99	1.25
Managed care administrative	25	0.07	0.13	0.19
Information technology	48	0.06	0.11	0.18
Housekeeping, maintenance, security	24	0.04	0.14	0.25
Medical receptionists	117	0.67	0.90	1.21
Medical secretaries, transcribers	106	0.33	0.53	0.94
Medical records	104	0.24	0.36	0.51
Other administrative support	47	0.07	0.24	0.53
Registered nurses	72	0.15	0.29	0.62
Licensed practical nurses	47	0.12	0.29	0.50
Medical assistants, nurse aides	98	0.33	0.60	1.02
Clinical laboratory	9	*	*	*
Radiology and imaging	112	0.34	0.46	0.59
Other medical support services	54	0.24	0.39	0.82
Total employed support staff	122	4.09	4.89	6.12
Total contracted support staff	49	0.10	0.20	0.35
Total support staff	122	4.16	4.97	6.21

Table 19b. Staff Cost per FTE Physician

		Orthopedic Surgery		
	Count	25th %tile	Median	75th %tile
General administrative	114	$ 12,014	$ 17,973	$ 22,352
Business office	116	$ 19,443	$ 24,397	$ 33,248
Managed care administrative	25	$ 2,274	$ 4,142	$ 6,525
Information technology	49	$ 2,474	$ 3,628	$ 5,942
Housekeeping, maintenance, security	27	$ 514	$ 2,818	$ 4,679
Medical receptionists	114	$ 13,481	$ 19,984	$ 27,377
Medical secretaries, transcribers	102	$ 9,105	$ 14,336	$ 26,715
Medical records	101	$ 4,415	$ 6,871	$ 10,952
Other administrative support	45	$ 1,716	$ 5,129	$ 10,191
Registered nurses	71	$ 6,304	$ 11,244	$ 21,876
Licensed practical nurses	45	$ 4,144	$ 8,129	$ 16,716
Medical assistants, nurse aides	94	$ 8,504	$ 15,105	$ 31,311
Clinical laboratory	9	*	*	*
Radiology and imaging	109	$ 11,759	$ 15,008	$ 18,459
Other medical support services	53	$ 7,451	$ 12,304	$ 28,120
Total employed support staff cost	121	$ 118,050	$ 141,441	$ 185,011
Total employed support staff benefits	116	$ 26,070	$ 34,742	$ 46,628
Total contracted support staff	58	$ 2,225	$ 6,549	$ 11,899
Total support staff cost	122	$ 148,872	$ 183,497	$ 227,297

TABLE 19 ■ Continued

Table 19c. Staff Cost As a Percent of Total Medical Revenue

Orthopedic Surgery

	Count	25th %tile	Median	75th %tile
General administrative	114	1.60%	2.13%	2.70%
Business office	116	2.37%	3.19%	4.05%
Managed care administrative	25	0.32%	0.52%	0.87%
Information technology	49	0.28%	0.43%	0.70%
Housekeeping, maintenance, security	27	0.07%	0.32%	0.49%
Medical receptionists	114	1.60%	2.66%	3.72%
Medical secretaries, transcribers	102	1.14%	1.82%	3.27%
Medical records	101	0.54%	0.86%	1.18%
Other administrative support	45	0.22%	0.63%	1.61%
Registered nurses	71	0.80%	1.65%	2.63%
Licensed practical nurses	45	0.47%	1.00%	1.97%
Medical assistants, nurse aides	94	1.05%	2.24%	3.69%
Clinical laboratory	9	*	*	*
Radiology and imaging	109	1.40%	1.73%	2.47%
Other medical support services	53	0.95%	1.58%	3.13%
Total employed support staff cost	121	15.37%	18.27%	21.03%
Total employed support staff benefits	116	3.45%	4.37%	5.39%
Total contracted support staff	58	0.24%	0.91%	1.70%
Total support staff cost	122	20.32%	23.43%	26.48%

Table 19d. FTE Staff per FTE Physician (Staff Categories)

Orthopedic Surgery

	Count	25th %tile	Median	75th %tile
Administrative and Business Staff per FTE Physician	121	1.01	1.29	1.67
Front Office Staff per FTE Physician	120	1.48	1.98	2.51
Clinical Staff per FTE Physician	113	0.67	1.00	1.37
Ancillary Service Staff per FTE Physician	116	0.45	0.61	0.89

Table 19e. Staff Cost per FTE Physician (Staff Categories)

Orthopedic Surgery

	Count	25th %tile	Median	75th %tile
Administrative and Business Staff Salary per FTE Physician	119	$ 35,619	$ 44,522	$ 57,538
Front Office Staff Salary per FTE Physician	117	$ 33,863	$ 45,812	$ 59,583
Clinical Staff Salary per FTE Physician	110	$ 19,097	$ 30,578	$ 44,720
Ancillary Service Staff Salary per FTE Physician	113	$ 14,777	$ 20,080	$ 30,157

Table 19f. Staff Cost As a Percent of Total Medical Revenue (Staff Categories)

Orthopedic Surgery

	Count	25th %tile	Median	75th %tile
Administrative and Business Staff Salary As % of Total Medical Revenue	119	4.46%	5.76%	7.09%
Front Office Staff Salary As % of Total Medical Revenue	117	4.52%	5.71%	7.40%
Clinical Staff Salary As % of Total Medical Revenue	110	2.54%	3.73%	5.12%
Ancillary Service Staff Salary As % of Total Medical Revenue	113	1.87%	2.50%	3.79%

TABLE 20 — Otorhinolaryngology, Not Hospital/Integrated Delivery System Owned

Table 20a. FTE Staff per FTE Physician

	Count	**Otorhinolaryngology 25th %tile**	**Median**	**75th %tile**
General administrative	16	0.17	0.23	0.27
Business office	16	0.78	1.02	1.38
Managed care administrative	2	*	*	*
Information technology	3	*	*	*
Housekeeping, maintenance, security	0	*	*	*
Medical receptionists	17	0.87	1.25	1.63
Medical secretaries, transcribers	10	0.15	0.26	0.52
Medical records	11	0.13	0.36	0.43
Other administrative support	5	*	*	*
Registered nurses	13	0.19	0.29	0.61
Licensed practical nurses	12	0.27	0.49	1.15
Medical assistants, nurse aides	16	0.45	0.63	1.13
Clinical laboratory	2	*	*	*
Radiology and imaging	0	*	*	*
Other medical support services	9	*	*	*
Total employed support staff	17	3.91	4.50	5.00
Total contracted support staff	6	*	*	*
Total support staff	17	4.03	4.69	5.02

Table 20b. Staff Cost per FTE Physician

	Count	**Otorhinolaryngology 25th %tile**	**Median**	**75th %tile**
General administrative	16	$ 9,728	$ 12,069	$ 17,694
Business office	16	$ 20,348	$ 27,043	$ 35,218
Managed care administrative	2	*	*	*
Information technology	3	*	*	*
Housekeeping, maintenance, security	0	*	*	*
Medical receptionists	17	$ 16,721	$ 24,258	$ 30,346
Medical secretaries, transcribers	10	$ 4,155	$ 6,328	$ 12,810
Medical records	11	$ 2,313	$ 4,848	$ 9,253
Other administrative support	6	*	*	*
Registered nurses	13	$ 6,575	$ 16,402	$ 24,548
Licensed practical nurses	12	$ 6,634	$ 13,098	$ 32,628
Medical assistants, nurse aides	16	$ 6,934	$ 13,599	$ 28,015
Clinical laboratory	2	*	*	*
Radiology and imaging	0	*	*	*
Other medical support services	9	*	*	*
Total employed support staff cost	17	$ 104,960	$ 125,206	$ 137,698
Total employed support staff benefits	15	$ 20,880	$ 28,763	$ 31,116
Total contracted support staff	11	$ 1,003	$ 2,599	$ 10,511
Total support staff cost	17	$ 137,854	$ 152,828	$ 163,072

TABLE 20 ◼ Continued

Table 20c. Staff Cost As a Percent of Total Medical Revenue

		Otorhinolaryngology		
	Count	25th %tile	Median	75th %tile
General administrative	16	1.56%	2.00%	2.49%
Business office	16	3.33%	4.07%	4.77%
Managed care administrative	2	*	*	*
Information technology	3	*	*	*
Housekeeping, maintenance, security	0	*	*	*
Medical receptionists	17	2.51%	3.05%	4.30%
Medical secretaries, transcribers	10	0.69%	0.98%	2.07%
Medical records	11	0.36%	0.45%	1.25%
Other administrative support	6	*	*	*
Registered nurses	13	0.90%	2.25%	3.10%
Licensed practical nurses	12	1.03%	2.35%	5.39%
Medical assistants, nurse aides	16	1.19%	2.37%	3.52%
Clinical laboratory	2	*	*	*
Radiology and imaging	0	*	*	*
Other medical support services	9	*	*	*
Total employed support staff cost	17	16.02%	17.68%	20.33%
Total employed support staff benefits	15	3.59%	3.92%	5.25%
Total contracted support staff	11	0.15%	0.30%	1.48%
Total support staff cost	17	19.88%	21.67%	23.37%

Table 20d. FTE Staff per FTE Physician (Staff Categories)

		Otorhinolaryngology		
	Count	25th %tile	Median	75th %tile
Administrative and Business Staff per FTE Physician	17	1.00	1.18	1.54
Front Office Staff per FTE Physician	17	1.20	1.69	2.07
Clinical Staff per FTE Physician	17	1.22	1.44	1.78
Ancillary Service Staff per FTE Physician	10	0.21	0.29	0.37

Table 20e. Staff Cost per FTE Physician (Staff Categories)

		Otorhinolaryngology		
	Count	25th %tile	Median	75th %tile
Administrative and Business Staff Salary per FTE Physician	17	$ 31,698	$ 36,284	$ 52,222
Front Office Staff Salary per FTE Physician	17	$ 24,686	$ 30,729	$ 44,958
Clinical Staff Salary per FTE Physician	17	$ 33,520	$ 42,901	$ 51,127
Ancillary Service Staff Salary per FTE Physician	10	$ 4,792	$ 9,804	$ 16,133

Table 20f. Staff Cost As a Percent of Total Medical Revenue (Staff Categories)

		Otorhinolaryngology		
	Count	25th %tile	Median	75th %tile
Administrative and Business Staff Salary As % of Total Medical Revenue	17	5.12%	5.78%	7.09%
Front Office Staff Salary As % of Total Medical Revenue	17	3.97%	4.90%	6.15%
Clinical Staff Salary As % of Total Medical Revenue	17	4.88%	6.42%	7.32%
Ancillary Service Staff Salary As % of Total Medical Revenue	10	0.70%	1.11%	2.28%

TABLE 21 — Pathology, Not Hospital/Integrated Delivery System Owned

Table 21a. FTE Staff per FTE Physician

	Count	25th %tile	Median	75th %tile
General administrative	10	0.21	0.34	0.46
Business office	8	*	*	*
Managed care administrative	0	*	*	*
Information technology	3	*	*	*
Housekeeping, maintenance, security	1	*	*	*
Medical receptionists	2	*	*	*
Medical secretaries, transcribers	5	*	*	*
Medical records	0	*	*	*
Other administrative support	4	*	*	*
Registered nurses	0	*	*	*
Licensed practical nurses	0	*	*	*
Medical assistants, nurse aides	0	*	*	*
Clinical laboratory	8	*	*	*
Radiology and imaging	0	*	*	*
Other medical support services	2	*	*	*
Total employed support staff	9	*	*	*
Total contracted support staff	6	*	*	*
Total support staff	11	0.82	2.17	3.38

Table 21b. Staff Cost per FTE Physician

	Count	25th %tile	Median	75th %tile
General administrative	10	$11,836	$23,710	$38,635
Business office	8	*	*	*
Managed care administrative	0	*	*	*
Information technology	3	*	*	*
Housekeeping, maintenance, security	1	*	*	*
Medical receptionists	2	*	*	*
Medical secretaries, transcribers	5	*	*	*
Medical records	0	*	*	*
Other administrative support	4	*	*	*
Registered nurses	0	*	*	*
Licensed practical nurses	0	*	*	*
Medical assistants, nurse aides	0	*	*	*
Clinical laboratory	8	*	*	*
Radiology and imaging	0	*	*	*
Other medical support services	2	*	*	*
Total employed support staff cost	10	$34,871	$94,127	$148,267
Total employed support staff benefits	9	*	*	*
Total contracted support staff	6	*	*	*
Total support staff cost	11	$32,367	$110,055	$184,121

TABLE 21 ■ Continued

Table 21c. Staff Cost As a Percent of Total Medical Revenue

		Pathology		
	Count	25th %tile	Median	75th %tile
General administrative	10	1.84%	3.74%	6.03%
Business office	8	*	*	*
Managed care administrative	0	*	*	*
Information technology	3	*	*	*
Housekeeping, maintenance, security	1	*	*	*
Medical receptionists	2	*	*	*
Medical secretaries, transcribers	5	*	*	*
Medical records	0	*	*	*
Other administrative support	4	*	*	*
Registered nurses	0	*	*	*
Licensed practical nurses	0	*	*	*
Medical assistants, nurse aides	0	*	*	*
Clinical laboratory	8	*	*	*
Radiology and imaging	0	*	*	*
Other medical support services	2	*	*	*
Total employed support staff cost	10	6.63%	16.38%	18.71%
Total employed support staff benefits	9	*	*	*
Total contracted support staff	6	*	*	*
Total support staff cost	11	6.07%	18.62%	26.22%

Table 21d. FTE Staff per FTE Physician (Staff Categories)

		Pathology		
	Count	25th %tile	Median	75th %tile
Administrative and Business Staff per FTE Physician	11	0.36	0.96	1.28
Front Office Staff per FTE Physician	9	*	*	*
Clinical Staff per FTE Physician	0	*	*	*
Ancillary Service Staff per FTE Physician	8	*	*	*

Table 21e. Staff Cost per FTE Physician (Staff Categories)

		Pathology		
	Count	25th %tile	Median	75th %tile
Administrative and Business Staff Salary per FTE Physician	11	$ 21,127	$ 36,182	$ 46,459
Front Office Staff Salary per FTE Physician	9	*	*	*
Clinical Staff Salary per FTE Physician	0	*	*	*
Ancillary Service Staff Salary per FTE Physician	8	*	*	*

Table 21f. Staff Cost As a Percent of Total Medical Revenue (Staff Categories)

		Pathology		
	Count	25th %tile	Median	75th %tile
Administrative and Business Staff Salary As % of Total Medical Revenue	11	3.87%	6.49%	9.53%
Front Office Staff Salary As % of Total Medical Revenue	9	*	*	*
Clinical Staff Salary As % of Total Medical Revenue	0	*	*	*
Ancillary Service Staff Salary As % of Total Medical Revenue	8	*	*	*

TABLE 22 — Pediatrics, Not Hospital/Integrated Delivery System Owned

Table 22a. FTE Staff per FTE Physician

		Pediatrics		
	Count	25th %tile	Median	75th %tile
General administrative	20	0.15	0.22	0.33
Business office	21	0.52	0.69	0.78
Managed care administrative	9	*	*	*
Information technology	1	*	*	*
Housekeeping, maintenance, security	2	*	*	*
Medical receptionists	22	0.73	0.97	1.30
Medical secretaries, transcribers	7	*	*	*
Medical records	14	0.13	0.35	0.50
Other administrative support	7	*	*	*
Registered nurses	20	0.25	0.57	0.79
Licensed practical nurses	18	0.15	0.27	0.82
Medical assistants, nurse aides	19	0.37	0.83	1.07
Clinical laboratory	5	*	*	*
Radiology and imaging	3	*	*	*
Other medical support services	1	*	*	*
Total employed support staff	22	3.50	4.04	4.45
Total contracted support staff	5	*	*	*
Total support staff	22	3.50	4.05	4.48

Table 22b. Staff Cost per FTE Physician

		Pediatrics		
	Count	25th %tile	Median	75th %tile
General administrative	19	$ 9,316	$ 15,638	$ 19,263
Business office	20	$ 13,216	$ 18,948	$ 27,212
Managed care administrative	9	*	*	*
Information technology	1	*	*	*
Housekeeping, maintenance, security	2	*	*	*
Medical receptionists	21	$ 15,799	$ 21,649	$ 27,218
Medical secretaries, transcribers	7	*	*	*
Medical records	13	$ 2,171	$ 4,555	$ 7,274
Other administrative support	7	*	*	*
Registered nurses	20	$ 6,343	$ 17,198	$ 30,746
Licensed practical nurses	18	$ 5,358	$ 10,545	$ 20,835
Medical assistants, nurse aides	19	$ 8,115	$ 15,388	$ 23,920
Clinical laboratory	6	*	*	*
Radiology and imaging	3	*	*	*
Other medical support services	1	*	*	*
Total employed support staff cost	22	$ 93,420	$ 116,949	$ 124,134
Total employed support staff benefits	22	$ 17,836	$ 22,995	$ 25,941
Total contracted support staff	11	$ 934	$ 1,603	$ 6,629
Total support staff cost	22	$ 115,926	$ 134,527	$ 155,861

TABLE 22 ■ Continued

Table 22c. Staff Cost As a Percent of Total Medical Revenue

		Pediatrics		
	Count	25th %tile	Median	75th %tile
General administrative	19	2.01%	2.68%	3.82%
Business office	20	2.69%	3.89%	5.39%
Managed care administrative	9	*	*	*
Information technology	1	*	*	*
Housekeeping, maintenance, security	2	*	*	*
Medical receptionists	21	3.22%	4.58%	5.47%
Medical secretaries, transcribers	7	*	*	*
Medical records	13	0.43%	0.97%	1.53%
Other administrative support	7	*	*	*
Registered nurses	20	1.61%	3.11%	6.32%
Licensed practical nurses	18	1.13%	2.23%	4.12%
Medical assistants, nurse aides	19	1.57%	3.21%	5.29%
Clinical laboratory	6	*	*	*
Radiology and imaging	3	*	*	*
Other medical support services	1	*	*	*
Total employed support staff cost	22	19.85%	22.69%	25.02%
Total employed support staff benefits	22	3.85%	4.57%	5.76%
Total contracted support staff	11	0.19%	0.40%	1.66%
Total support staff cost	22	25.76%	28.01%	30.99%

Table 22d. FTE Staff per FTE Physician (Staff Categories)

		Pediatrics		
	Count	25th %tile	Median	75th %tile
Administrative and Business Staff per FTE Physician	22	0.72	0.99	1.25
Front Office Staff per FTE Physician	22	1.15	1.36	1.69
Clinical Staff per FTE Physician	21	1.26	1.76	1.94
Ancillary Service Staff per FTE Physician	6	*	*	*

Table 22e. Staff Cost per FTE Physician (Staff Categories)

		Pediatrics		
	Count	25th %tile	Median	75th %tile
Administrative and Business Staff Salary per FTE Physician	21	$ 25,147	$ 33,308	$ 43,274
Front Office Staff Salary per FTE Physician	21	$ 21,931	$ 27,659	$ 35,015
Clinical Staff Salary per FTE Physician	21	$ 35,179	$ 46,750	$ 54,092
Ancillary Service Staff Salary per FTE Physician	7	*	*	*

Table 22f. Staff Cost As a Percent of Total Medical Revenue (Staff Categories)

		Pediatrics		
	Count	25th %tile	Median	75th %tile
Administrative and Business Staff Salary As % of Total Medical Revenue	21	5.37%	7.62%	8.11%
Front Office Staff Salary As % of Total Medical Revenue	21	4.26%	6.02%	7.21%
Clinical Staff Salary As % of Total Medical Revenue	21	7.48%	8.93%	11.08%
Ancillary Service Staff Salary As % of Total Medical Revenue	7	*	*	*

TABLE 23 — Pediatrics, Hospital/Integrated Delivery System Owned

Table 23a. FTE Staff per FTE Physician

	Pediatrics (Hospital / IDS Owned)			
	Count	25th %tile	Median	75th %tile
General administrative	14	0.13	0.23	0.27
Business office	18	0.30	0.61	1.02
Managed care administrative	3	*	*	*
Information technology	1	*	*	*
Housekeeping, maintenance, security	2	*	*	*
Medical receptionists	13	0.65	1.16	1.43
Medical secretaries, transcribers	7	*	*	*
Medical records	8	*	*	*
Other administrative support	10	0.22	0.53	1.54
Registered nurses	18	0.48	0.80	1.16
Licensed practical nurses	19	0.20	0.43	0.85
Medical assistants, nurse aides	15	0.21	0.28	0.48
Clinical laboratory	6	*	*	*
Radiology and imaging	0	*	*	*
Other medical support services	4	*	*	*
Total employed support staff	20	3.48	4.15	5.04
Total contracted support staff	5	*	*	*
Total support staff	23	3.50	4.14	4.92

Table 23b. Staff Cost per FTE Physician

	Pediatrics (Hospital / IDS Owned)			
	Count	25th %tile	Median	75th %tile
General administrative	10	$ 4,874	$ 12,264	$ 14,123
Business office	14	$ 9,849	$ 11,653	$ 27,237
Managed care administrative	2	*	*	*
Information technology	0	*	*	*
Housekeeping, maintenance, security	1	*	*	*
Medical receptionists	9	*	*	*
Medical secretaries, transcribers	6	*	*	*
Medical records	5	*	*	*
Other administrative support	9	*	*	*
Registered nurses	14	$ 17,551	$ 25,856	$ 42,761
Licensed practical nurses	15	$ 4,246	$ 10,516	$ 22,935
Medical assistants, nurse aides	12	$ 4,544	$ 6,865	$ 8,733
Clinical laboratory	5	*	*	*
Radiology and imaging	0	*	*	*
Other medical support services	3	*	*	*
Total employed support staff cost	22	$ 80,676	$ 106,038	$ 124,460
Total employed support staff benefits	22	$ 12,281	$ 19,280	$ 23,035
Total contracted support staff	13	$ 326	$ 1,300	$ 6,847
Total support staff cost	23	$ 105,122	$ 127,001	$ 148,579

TABLE 23 ■ Continued

Table 23c. Staff Cost As a Percent of Total Medical Revenue

Pediatrics (Hospital / IDS Owned)

	Count	25th %tile	Median	75th %tile
General administrative	10	1.02%	2.40%	4.30%
Business office	14	2.42%	3.30%	4.76%
Managed care administrative	2	*	*	*
Information technology	0	*	*	*
Housekeeping, maintenance, security	1	*	*	*
Medical receptionists	9	*	*	*
Medical secretaries, transcribers	6	*	*	*
Medical records	5	*	*	*
Other administrative support	9	*	*	*
Registered nurses	14	4.47%	5.84%	8.52%
Licensed practical nurses	15	0.99%	2.71%	5.29%
Medical assistants, nurse aides	12	1.01%	1.38%	2.27%
Clinical laboratory	5	*	*	*
Radiology and imaging	0	*	*	*
Other medical support services	3	*	*	*
Total employed support staff cost	22	20.74%	24.04%	32.01%
Total employed support staff benefits	22	3.88%	4.58%	5.19%
Total contracted support staff	13	0.09%	0.36%	1.41%
Total support staff cost	23	24.74%	29.75%	37.46%

Table 23d. FTE Staff per FTE Physician (Staff Categories)

Pediatrics (Hospital / IDS Owned)

	Count	25th %tile	Median	75th %tile
Administrative and Business Staff per FTE Physician	19	0.50	0.67	1.27
Front Office Staff per FTE Physician	19	1.06	1.33	1.85
Clinical Staff per FTE Physician	19	1.06	1.56	2.09
Ancillary Service Staff per FTE Physician	8	*	*	*

Table 23e. Staff Cost per FTE Physician (Staff Categories)

Pediatrics (Hospital / IDS Owned)

	Count	25th %tile	Median	75th %tile
Administrative and Business Staff Salary per FTE Physician	15	$ 12,265	$ 18,246	$ 40,898
Front Office Staff Salary per FTE Physician	15	$ 23,413	$ 31,408	$ 38,013
Clinical Staff Salary per FTE Physician	15	$ 32,943	$ 42,169	$ 67,214
Ancillary Service Staff Salary per FTE Physician	6	*	*	*

Table 23f. Staff Cost As a Percent of Total Medical Revenue (Staff Categories)

Pediatrics (Hospital / IDS Owned)

	Count	25th %tile	Median	75th %tile
Administrative and Business Staff Salary As % of Total Medical Revenue	15	3.75%	4.13%	7.80%
Front Office Staff Salary As % of Total Medical Revenue	15	5.43%	7.95%	8.53%
Clinical Staff Salary As % of Total Medical Revenue	15	8.16%	10.05%	14.91%
Ancillary Service Staff Salary As % of Total Medical Revenue	6	*	*	*

TABLE 24 ■ Radiology, Not Hospital/Integrated Delivery System Owned

Table 24a. FTE Staff per FTE Physician

	Count	Radiology 25th %tile	Median	75th %tile
General administrative	20	0.13	0.20	0.39
Business office	18	0.84	1.14	1.41
Managed care administrative	4	*	*	*
Information technology	9	*	*	*
Housekeeping, maintenance, security	2	*	*	*
Medical receptionists	13	0.42	0.56	0.76
Medical secretaries, transcribers	14	0.09	0.21	0.26
Medical records	12	0.09	0.22	0.36
Other administrative support	6	*	*	*
Registered nurses	3	*	*	*
Licensed practical nurses	0	*	*	*
Medical assistants, nurse aides	0	*	*	*
Clinical laboratory	0	*	*	*
Radiology and imaging	16	0.50	1.15	1.85
Other medical support services	3	*	*	*
Total employed support staff	21	1.23	2.92	4.81
Total contracted support staff	12	0.04	0.08	0.26
Total support staff	21	1.44	2.92	4.85

Table 24b. Staff Cost per FTE Physician

	Count	Radiology 25th %tile	Median	75th %tile
General administrative	19	$ 7,052	$ 16,474	$ 22,410
Business office	17	$ 21,576	$ 28,736	$ 40,556
Managed care administrative	4	*	*	*
Information technology	8	*	*	*
Housekeeping, maintenance, security	3	*	*	*
Medical receptionists	12	$ 9,986	$ 13,057	$ 17,698
Medical secretaries, transcribers	13	$ 2,189	$ 6,430	$ 8,769
Medical records	11	$ 2,112	$ 4,837	$ 6,235
Other administrative support	6	*	*	*
Registered nurses	3	*	*	*
Licensed practical nurses	0	*	*	*
Medical assistants, nurse aides	0	*	*	*
Clinical laboratory	0	*	*	*
Radiology and imaging	15	$ 16,016	$ 33,488	$ 63,537
Other medical support services	2	*	*	*
Total employed support staff cost	21	$ 39,595	$ 102,414	$ 148,876
Total employed support staff benefits	18	$ 12,754	$ 18,197	$ 34,317
Total contracted support staff	14	$ 815	$ 3,867	$ 7,993
Total support staff cost	21	$ 61,202	$ 120,941	$ 184,314

TABLE 24 ■ Continued

Table 24c. Staff Cost As a Percent of Total Medical Revenue

	Count	25th %tile	Median	75th %tile
		\multicolumn{3}{c}{Radiology}	
General administrative	19	1.26%	1.89%	2.49%
Business office	17	2.72%	3.83%	5.68%
Managed care administrative	4	*	*	*
Information technology	8	*	*	*
Housekeeping, maintenance, security	3	*	*	*
Medical receptionists	12	0.79%	1.75%	2.68%
Medical secretaries, transcribers	13	0.40%	0.72%	1.07%
Medical records	11	0.26%	0.61%	0.75%
Other administrative support	6	*	*	*
Registered nurses	3	*	*	*
Licensed practical nurses	0	*	*	*
Medical assistants, nurse aides	0	c	*	*
Clinical laboratory	0	*	*	*
Radiology and imaging	15	2.69%	4.49%	6.84%
Other medical support services	2	*	*	*
Total employed support staff cost	21	6.14%	13.91%	16.42%
Total employed support staff benefits	18	1.98%	2.64%	4.84%
Total contracted support staff	14	0.12%	0.56%	1.10%
Total support staff cost	21	10.24%	16.03%	22.09%

Table 24d. FTE Staff per FTE Physician (Staff Categories)

	Count	25th %tile	Median	75th %tile
		\multicolumn{3}{c}{Radiology}	
Administrative and Business Staff per FTE Physician	20	0.93	1.42	1.76
Front Office Staff per FTE Physician	15	0.40	1.10	1.44
Clinical Staff per FTE Physician	3	*	*	*
Ancillary Service Staff per FTE Physician	17	0.38	1.13	1.74

Table 24e. Staff Cost per FTE Physician (Staff Categories)

	Count	25th %tile	Median	75th %tile
		\multicolumn{3}{c}{Radiology}	
Administrative and Business Staff Salary per FTE Physician	19	$32,706	$49,522	$67,784
Front Office Staff Salary per FTE Physician	14	$10,484	$25,999	$34,774
Clinical Staff Salary per FTE Physician	3	*	*	*
Ancillary Service Staff Salary per FTE Physician	16	$14,694	$29,705	$62,518

Table 24f. Staff Cost As a Percent of Total Medical Revenue (Staff Categories)

	Count	25th %tile	Median	75th %tile
		\multicolumn{3}{c}{Radiology}	
Administrative and Business Staff Salary As % of Total Medical Revenue	19	4.32%	6.29%	7.58%
Front Office Staff Salary As % of Total Medical Revenue	14	1.43%	3.08%	4.77%
Clinical Staff Salary As % of Total Medical Revenue	3	*	*	*
Ancillary Service Staff Salary As % of Total Medical Revenue	16	2.67%	3.96%	6.72%

TABLE 25 — Surgery: Cardiovascular, Not Hospital/Integrated Delivery System Owned

Table 25a. FTE Staff per FTE Physician

		Surgery: Cardiovascular		
	Count	25th %tile	Median	75th %tile
General administrative	13	0.12	0.17	0.26
Business office	15	0.40	0.50	0.60
Managed care administrative	2	*	*	*
Information technology	7	*	*	*
Housekeeping, maintenance, security	1	*	*	*
Medical receptionists	16	0.23	0.33	0.53
Medical secretaries, transcribers	13	0.16	0.32	0.47
Medical records	8	*	*	*
Other administrative support	6	*	*	*
Registered nurses	13	0.32	0.50	0.73
Licensed practical nurses	3	*	*	*
Medical assistants, nurse aides	7	*	*	*
Clinical laboratory	0	*	*	*
Radiology and imaging	5	*	*	*
Other medical support services	5	*	*	*
Total employed support staff	16	1.46	2.34	3.20
Total contracted support staff	6	*	*	*
Total support staff	16	1.52	2.34	3.33

Table 25b. Staff Cost per FTE Physician

		Surgery: Cardiovascular		
	Count	25th %tile	Median	75th %tile
General administrative	11	$ 13,818	$ 17,333	$ 18,727
Business office	12	$ 10,495	$ 14,410	$ 19,755
Managed care administrative	2	*	*	*
Information technology	6	*	*	*
Housekeeping, maintenance, security	1	*	*	*
Medical receptionists	13	$ 4,178	$ 6,356	$ 11,927
Medical secretaries, transcribers	11	$ 6,521	$ 9,503	$ 13,333
Medical records	6	*	*	*
Other administrative support	5	*	*	*
Registered nurses	10	$ 10,615	$ 22,317	$ 27,259
Licensed practical nurses	3	*	*	*
Medical assistants, nurse aides	7	*	*	*
Clinical laboratory	0	*	*	*
Radiology and imaging	4	*	*	*
Other medical support services	5	*	*	*
Total employed support staff cost	16	$ 56,704	$ 78,124	$ 118,021
Total employed support staff benefits	6	$ 12,875	$ 21,396	$ 34,375
Total contracted support staff	17	*	*	*
Total support staff cost	16	$ 71,276	$ 97,895	$ 153,337

TABLE 25 Continued

Table 25c. Staff Cost As a Percent of Total Medical Revenue

		Surgery: Cardiovascular		
	Count	25th %tile	Median	75th %tile
General administrative	11	1.60%	1.99%	2.39%
Business office	12	1.29%	1.97%	2.65%
Managed care administrative	2	*	*	*
Information technology	6	*	*	*
Housekeeping, maintenance, security	1	*	*	*
Medical receptionists	13	0.63%	0.86%	2.17%
Medical secretaries, transcribers	11	0.81%	1.27%	1.51%
Medical records	6	*	*	*
Other administrative support	5	*	*	*
Registered nurses	10	1.66%	2.33%	2.67%
Licensed practical nurses	3	*	*	*
Medical assistants, nurse aides	7	*	*	*
Clinical laboratory	0	*	*	*
Radiology and imaging	4	*	*	*
Other medical support services	5	*	*	*
Total employed support staff cost	16	6.79%	10.71%	14.32%
Total employed support staff benefits	16	1.72%	2.78%	3.84%
Total contracted support staff	7	*	*	*
Total support staff cost	16	9.58%	12.34%	18.57%

Table 25d. FTE Staff per FTE Physician (Staff Categories)

		Surgery: Cardiovascular		
	Count	25th %tile	Median	75th %tile
Administrative and Business Staff per FTE Physician	16	0.54	0.67	0.94
Front Office Staff per FTE Physician	16	0.56	0.75	1.22
Clinical Staff per FTE Physician	14	0.39	0.69	0.84
Ancillary Service Staff per FTE Physician	8	*	*	*

Table 25e. Staff Cost per FTE Physician (Staff Categories)

		Surgery: Cardiovascular		
	Count	25th %tile	Median	75th %tile
Administrative and Business Staff Salary per FTE Physician	13	$ 18,791	$ 29,859	$ 34,879
Front Office Staff Salary per FTE Physician	13	$ 14,121	$ 21,528	$ 32,960
Clinical Staff Salary per FTE Physician	11	$ 10,461	$ 24,890	$ 32,457
Ancillary Service Staff Salary per FTE Physician	7	*	*	*

Table 25f. Staff Cost As a Percent of Total Medical Revenue (Staff Categories)

		Surgery: Cardiovascular		
	Count	25th %tile	Median	75th %tile
Administrative and Business Staff Salary As % of Total Medical Revenue	13	2.72%	3.79%	4.90%
Front Office Staff Salary As % of Total Medical Revenue	13	2.03%	2.50%	3.71%
Clinical Staff Salary As % of Total Medical Revenue	11	1.73%	2.76%	3.85%
Ancillary Service Staff Salary As % of Total Medical Revenue	7	*	*	*

TABLE 26 — Surgery: General, Not Hospital/Integrated Delivery System Owned

Table 26a. FTE Staff per FTE Physician

		Surgery: General		
	Count	25th %tile	Median	75th %tile
General administrative	23	0.18	0.25	0.33
Business office	23	0.45	0.58	0.75
Managed care administrative	3	*	*	*
Information technology	5	*	*	*
Housekeeping, maintenance, security	1	*	*	*
Medical receptionists	23	0.36	0.50	0.75
Medical secretaries, transcribers	15	0.15	0.25	0.38
Medical records	17	0.12	0.16	0.27
Other administrative support	9	*	*	*
Registered nurses	16	0.19	0.42	0.60
Licensed practical nurses	14	0.13	0.25	0.49
Medical assistants, nurse aides	18	0.16	0.38	0.58
Clinical laboratory	1	*	*	*
Radiology and imaging	5	*	*	*
Other medical support services	3	*	*	*
Total employed support staff	23	2.50	2.89	3.25
Total contracted support staff	13	0.05	0.08	0.17
Total support staff	23	2.58	2.89	3.33

Table 26b. Staff Cost per FTE Physician

		Surgery: General		
	Count	25th %tile	Median	75th %tile
General administrative	22	$11,728	$15,069	$19,278
Business office	22	$14,612	$17,696	$23,390
Managed care administrative	3	*	*	*
Information technology	4	*	*	*
Housekeeping, maintenance, security	1	*	*	*
Medical receptionists	21	$8,012	$9,514	$14,357
Medical secretaries, transcribers	14	$4,043	$8,466	$14,458
Medical records	17	$2,329	$3,717	$5,429
Other administrative support	10	$4,528	$8,044	$10,394
Registered nurses	15	$6,000	$16,813	$23,125
Licensed practical nurses	13	$3,159	$4,246	$12,399
Medical assistants, nurse aides	18	$3,067	$10,204	$17,353
Clinical laboratory	1	*	*	*
Radiology and imaging	5	*	*	*
Other medical support services	3	*	*	*
Total employed support staff cost	23	$76,841	$92,784	$108,479
Total employed support staff benefits	23	$19,822	$24,078	$27,719
Total contracted support staff	16	$1,349	$3,068	$4,991
Total support staff cost	23	$103,284	$113,837	$137,000

TABLE 26 ■ Continued

Table 26c. Staff Cost As a Percent of Total Medical Revenue

		Surgery: General		
	Count	25th %tile	Median	75th %tile
General administrative	22	2.18%	2.81%	3.52%
Business office	22	2.77%	3.21%	3.70%
Managed care administrative	3	*	*	*
Information technology	4	*	*	*
Housekeeping, maintenance, security	1	*	*	*
Medical receptionists	21	1.36%	1.88%	2.89%
Medical secretaries, transcribers	14	0.53%	1.34%	2.45%
Medical records	17	0.43%	0.66%	1.01%
Other administrative support	10	0.52%	1.57%	2.31%
Registered nurses	15	0.93%	2.35%	4.05%
Licensed practical nurses	13	0.53%	0.95%	1.96%
Medical assistants, nurse aides	18	0.55%	2.10%	3.03%
Clinical laboratory	1	*	*	*
Radiology and imaging	5	*	*	*
Other medical support services	3	*	*	*
Total employed support staff cost	23	14.47%	16.82%	19.15%
Total employed support staff benefit	23	3.33%	4.30%	5.80%
Total contracted support staff	16	0.28%	0.50%	0.85%
Total support staff cost	23	18.38%	20.64%	24.62%

Table 26d. FTE Staff per FTE Physician (Staff Categories)

		Surgery: General		
	Count	25th %tile	Median	75th %tile
Administrative and Business Staff per FTE Physician	23	0.75	0.97	1.06
Front Office Staff per FTE Physician	23	0.73	1.00	1.31
Clinical Staff per FTE Physician	22	0.56	0.83	0.96
Ancillary Service Staff per FTE Physician	8	*	*	*

Table 26e. Staff Cost per FTE physician (Staff Categories)

		Surgery: General		
	Count	25th %tile	Median	75th %tile
Administrative and Business Staff Salary per FTE Physician	22	$ 29,500	$ 36,241	$ 41,351
Front Office Staff Salary per FTE Physician	22	$ 20,586	$ 25,581	$ 29,966
Clinical Staff Salary per FTE Physician	21	$ 19,498	$ 25,375	$ 30,449
Ancillary Service Staff Salary per FTE Physician	8	*	*	*

Table 26f. Staff Cost As a Percent of Total Medical Revenue (Staff Categories)

		Surgery: General		
	Count	25th %tile	Median	75th %tile
Administrative and Business Staff Salary As % of Total Medical Revenue	22	5.70%	6.42%	7.29%
Front Office Staff Salary As % of Total Medical Revenue	22	2.87%	4.70%	5.64%
Clinical Staff Salary As % of Total Medical Revenue	21	3.47%	4.26%	5.72%
Ancillary Service Staff Salary As % of Total Medical Revenue	8	*	*	*

TABLE 27 — All Multispecialty Practices

Table 27a. FTE Staff per FTE Physician

	Count	Surgery: Neurological 25th %tile	Median	75th %tile
General administrative	13	0.15	0.25	0.37
Business office	13	0.40	0.53	0.86
Managed care administrative	3	*	*	*
Information technology	3	*	*	*
Housekeeping, maintenance, security	1	*	*	*
Medical receptionists	13	0.35	0.50	0.88
Medical secretaries, transcribers	12	0.50	1.00	1.42
Medical records	11	0.13	0.22	0.29
Other administrative support	5	*	*	*
Registered nurses	6	*	*	*
Licensed practical nurses	6	*	*	*
Medical assistants, nurse aides	6	*	*	*
Clinical laboratory	0	*	*	*
Radiology and imaging	4	*	*	*
Other medical support services	3	*	*	*
Total employed support staff	13	2.94	3.50	3.99
Total contracted support staff	6	*	*	*
Total support staff	13	3.00	3.60	3.99

Table 27b. Staff Cost per FTE Physician

	Count	Surgery: Neurological 25th %tile	Median	75th %tile
General administrative	13	$11,607	$18,307	$25,272
Business office	13	$13,672	$16,371	$23,371
Managed care administrative	4	*	*	*
Information technology	4	*	*	*
Housekeeping, maintenance, security	2	*	*	*
Medical receptionists	12	$8,006	$8,978	$23,393
Medical secretaries, transcribers	11	$14,364	$35,000	$46,352
Medical records	10	$1,854	$3,117	$4,602
Other administrative support	5	*	*	*
Registered nurses	6	*	*	*
Licensed practical nurses	6	*	*	*
Medical assistants, nurse aides	6	*	*	*
Clinical laboratory	0	*	*	*
Radiology and imaging	4	*	*	*
Other medical support services	3	*	*	*
Total employed support staff cost	13	$84,520	$111,294	$138,560
Total employed support staff benefits	12	$26,477	$29,045	$50,978
Total contracted support staff	8	*	*	*
Total support staff cost	13	$111,693	$149,609	$184,015

TABLE 27 ■ Continued

Table 27c. Staff Cost As a Percent of Total Medical Revenue

	Count	Surgery: Neurological 25th %tile	Median	75th %tile
General administrative	13	1.56%	1.91%	2.72%
Business office	13	1.72%	2.14%	2.88%
Managed care administrative	4	*	*	*
Information technology	4	*	*	*
Housekeeping, maintenance, security	2	*	*	*
Medical receptionists	12	1.06%	1.27%	2.38%
Medical secretaries, transcribers	11	1.48%	4.64%	6.07%
Medical records	10	0.26%	0.43%	0.60%
Other administrative support	5	*	*	*
Registered nurses	6	*	*	*
Licensed practical nurses	6	*	*	*
Medical assistants, nurse aides	6	*	*	*
Clinical laboratory	0	*	*	*
Radiology and imaging	4	*	*	*
Other medical support services	3	*	*	*
Total employed support staff cost	13	11.97%	13.29%	15.54%
Total employed support staff benefits	12	3.37%	3.71%	5.65%
Total contracted support staff	8	*	*	*
Total support staff cost	13	15.99	17.90	21.99

Table 27d. FTE Staff per FTE Physician (Staff Categories)

	Count	Surgery: Neurological 25th %tile	Median	75th %tile
Administrative and Business Staff per FTE Physician	13	0.71	0.83	1.25
Front Office Staff per FTE Physician	13	1.27	1.75	2.10
Clinical Staff per FTE Physician	10	0.42	0.94	1.07
Ancillary Service Staff per FTE Physician	6	*	*	*

Table 27e. Staff Cost per FTE Physician (Staff Categories)

	Count	Surgery: Neurological 25th %tile	Median	75th %tile
Administrative and Business Staff Salary per FTE Physician	13	$ 29,951	$ 36,128	$ 56,603
Front Office Staff Salary per FTE Physician	12	$ 30,585	$ 48,072	$ 56,963
Clinical Staff Salary per FTE Physician	10	$ 7,765	$ 28,516	$ 48,659
Ancillary Service Staff Salary per FTE Physician	6	*	*	*

Table 27f. Staff Cost As a Percent of Total Medical Revenue (Staff Categories)

	Count	Surgery: Neurological 25th %tile	Median	75th %tile
Administrative and Business Staff Salary As % of Total Medical Revenue	13	3.68%	5.01%	6.83%
Front Office Staff Salary As % of Total Medical Revenue	12	3.81%	6.09%	7.61%
Clinical Staff Salary As % of Total Medical Revenue	10	1.21%	2.67%	4.97%
Ancillary Service Staff Salary As % of Total Medical Revenue	6	*	*	*

TABLE 28 — Urology, Not Hospital/Integrated Delivery System Owned

Table 28a. FTE Staff per FTE Physician

		Urology		
	Count	25th %tile	Median	75th %tile
General administrative	30	0.21	0.29	0.33
Business office	31	0.47	0.68	0.81
Managed care administrative	1	*	*	*
Information technology	8	*	*	*
Housekeeping, maintenance, security	3	*	*	*
Medical receptionists	30	0.57	0.99	1.40
Medical secretaries, transcribers	23	0.23	0.33	0.63
Medical records	25	0.17	0.33	0.53
Other administrative support	13	0.20	0.31	0.55
Registered nurses	23	0.17	0.33	0.69
Licensed practical nurses	21	0.24	0.33	0.58
Medical assistants, nurse aides	27	0.27	0.60	0.99
Clinical laboratory	16	0.15	0.24	0.29
Radiology and imaging	16	0.07	0.12	0.26
Other medical support services	5	*	*	*
Total employed support staff	31	3.50	4.05	5.47
Total contracted support staff	10	0.18	0.24	0.53
Total support staff	31	3.56	4.20	5.47

Table 28b. Staff Cost per FTE Physician

		Urology		
	Count	25th %tile	Median	75th %tile
General administrative	30	$ 13,289	$ 19,244	$ 21,948
Business office	31	$ 13,173	$ 18,091	$ 23,531
Managed care administrative	1	*	*	*
Information technology	8	*	*	*
Housekeeping, maintenance, security	4	*	*	*
Medical receptionists	30	$ 12,553	$ 20,505	$ 28,377
Medical secretaries, transcribers	23	$ 6,514	$ 8,552	$ 18,050
Medical records	25	$ 2,942	$ 6,980	$ 10,153
Other administrative support	12	$ 5,842	$ 7,518	$ 8,044
Registered nurses	24	$ 6,796	$ 13,662	$ 24,136
Licensed practical nurses	20	$ 7,462	$ 10,551	$ 15,778
Medical assistants, nurse aides	27	$ 8,147	$ 14,632	$ 25,644
Clinical laboratory	16	$ 3,490	$ 5,330	$ 8,719
Radiology and imaging	16	$ 2,274	$ 4,863	$ 9,901
Other medical support services	5	*	*	*
Total employed support staff cost	31	$ 104,487	$ 119,853	$ 155,268
Total employed support staff benefits	30	$ 23,138	$ 28,558	$ 39,926
Total contracted support staff	12	$ 2,211	$ 3,444	$ 10,365
Total support staff cost	31	$ 133,798	$ 147,795	$ 199,607

TABLE 28 ■ Continued

Table 28c. Staff Cost As a Percent of Total Medical Revenue

		Urology		
	Count	25th %tile	Median	75th %tile
General administrative	30	1.59%	2.26%	3.17%
Business office	31	1.84%	2.39%	3.06%
Managed care administrative	1	*	*	*
Information technology	8	*	*	*
Housekeeping, maintenance, security	4	*	*	*
Medical receptionists	30	1.88%	2.53%	3.86%
Medical secretaries, transcribers	23	0.93%	1.16%	2.13%
Medical records	25	0.41%	0.88%	1.10%
Other administrative support	12	0.84%	1.02%	1.15%
Registered nurses	24	1.01%	1.68%	3.17%
Licensed practical nurses	20	0.97%	1.37%	2.27%
Medical assistants, nurse aides	27	1.17%	1.89%	2.88%
Clinical laboratory	16	0.43%	0.72%	1.03%
Radiology and imaging	16	0.32%	0.64%	1.04%
Other medical support services	5	*	*	*
Total employed support staff cost	31	13.89%	15.80%	18.40%
Total employed support staff benefits	30	2.74%	4.01%	5.63%
Total contracted support staff	12	0.30%	0.41%	1.05%
Total support staff cost	31	17.84	20.13	23.16

Table 28d. FTE Staff per FTE Physician (Staff Categories)

		Urology		
	Count	25th %tile	Median	75th %tile
Administrative and Business Staff per FTE Physician	31	0.80	1.00	1.16
Front Office Staff per FTE Physician	31	1.30	1.70	1.97
Clinical Staff per FTE Physician	31	0.95	1.33	1.54
Ancillary Service Staff per FTE Physician	20	0.14	0.41	0.68

Table 28e. Staff Cost per FTE Physician (Staff Categories)

		Urology		
	Count	25th %tile	Median	75th %tile
Administrative and Business Staff Salary per FTE Physician	31	$ 30,853	$ 37,480	$ 47,931
Front Office Staff Salary per FTE Physician	31	$ 29,160	$ 38,280	$ 51,833
Clinical Staff Salary per FTE Physician	31	$ 27,592	$ 36,714	$ 45,479
Ancillary Service Staff Salary per FTE Physician	20	$ 4,128	$ 11,619	$ 19,207

Table 28f. Staff Cost As a Percent of Total Medical Revenue (Staff Categories)

		Urology		
	Count	25th %tile	Median	75th %tile
Administrative and Business Staff Salary As % of Total Medical Revenue	31	3.34%	5.06%	5.96%
Front Office Staff Salary As % of Total Medical Revenue	31	3.76%	5.22%	6.47%
Clinical Staff Salary As % of Total Medical Revenue	31	4.09%	4.80%	5.56%
Ancillary Service Staff Salary As % of Total Medical Revenue	20	0.50%	1.25%	2.30%

Appendix IV
MGMA Benchmarks—
Better Performing Practices
Comparison Tables

Appendix IV provides the key staffing benchmarks to be used in Step 1—Benchmark the Current State, when comparing a practice's staffing to those of better performing medical practices. The data include benchmarks at the **staff category level** (front office staff, general and administrative staff, clinical support staff, and ancillary service staff), as well as the **staff job classification level** for five different medical practice types: multispecialty groups, cardiology, family practice, obstetrics and gynecology, and orthopedic Surgery.

The following tables are computed from the Medical Group Management Association (MGMA) *Performance and Practices of Successful Medical Groups: 2001 Report Based on 2000 Data.* This report is based on data from the MGMA Cost Survey and relates the financial measures to the medical group's management practices.

The MGMA *Performance and Practices of Successful Medical Groups Report* features benchmarks of better performing medical groups that have satisfied specified criteria in one of four qualifying "performance areas":

1. Profitability and Cost Management
2. Productivity, Capacity, and Staffing
3. Accounts Receivable and Collections
4. Managed Care Operations

The staffing tables in Appendix IV reflect the staffing ratios for practices that met the selection criteria for productivity, capacity, and staffing. To qualify as a "better performer" in this performance area, a practice needed to report greater than the median for in-house professional procedures per square foot and greater than the median for in-house professional gross charges per physician. The criteria indicate that better performing practices have higher levels of production and, at the same time, have the best use of available space (capacity).

Each table compares staffing for practices that met the better practice selection criteria (better performers) with the staffing for practices that did not meet the selection criteria (not a better performer). The statistics for each table are the same as those reported in Appendix III and are described in the Appendix III introduction.

TABLE 1 ■ All Multispecialty Practices

Table 1a. FTE Staff per FTE Physician

	Count	Not a Better Performer 25th %tile	Median	75th %tile	Count	Better Performer 25th %tile	Median	75th %tile
General administrative	246	0.17	0.25	0.36	50	0.20	0.30	0.40
Business office	249	0.49	0.71	0.91	51	0.63	0.89	1.16
Managed care administrative	88	0.03	0.09	0.21	21	0.03	0.13	0.29
Information technology	131	0.06	0.09	0.17	34	0.06	0.11	0.19
Housekeeping, maintenance, security	136	0.05	0.11	0.21	33	0.03	0.14	0.23
Medical receptionists	242	0.64	0.85	1.17	48	0.68	0.92	1.18
Medical secretaries, transcribers	208	0.15	0.26	0.40	38	0.10	0.22	0.46
Medical records	217	0.25	0.37	0.53	47	0.29	0.42	0.66
Other administrative support	133	0.07	0.15	0.39	24	0.04	0.06	0.31
Registered nurses	221	0.23	0.50	0.80	48	0.23	0.46	0.83
Licensed practical nurses	224	0.23	0.48	0.82	40	0.18	0.40	0.72
Medical assistants, nurse aides	228	0.34	0.59	0.86	46	0.42	0.71	1.02
Clinical laboratory	196	0.18	0.31	0.46	44	0.25	0.33	0.49
Radiology and imaging	193	0.12	0.20	0.34	46	0.15	0.26	0.38
Other medical support services	132	0.09	0.24	0.44	35	0.11	0.20	0.35
Total employed support staff	277	3.90	4.84	5.64	52	4.72	5.49	6.75
Total contracted support staff	104	0.07	0.14	0.26	24	0.06	0.18	0.31
Total support staff	280	3.97	4.89	5.78	52	4.72	5.55	6.78

Table 1b. Staff Cost per FTE Physician

	Count	Not a Better Performer 25th %tile	Median	75th %tile	Count	Better Performer 25th %tile	Median	75th %tile
General administrative	246	$ 9,852	$ 13,960	$ 19,279	50	$ 12,423	$ 15,965	$ 20,084
Business office	251	$ 12,327	$ 17,146	$ 22,238	50	$ 15,250	$ 20,796	$ 27,790
Managed care administrative	90	$ 1,150	$ 2,599	$ 5,338	21	$ 1,627	$ 5,093	$ 8,284
Information technology	132	$ 1,978	$ 3,468	$ 5,056	34	$ 2,270	$ 3,663	$ 5,842
Housekeeping, maintenance, security	140	$ 1,026	$ 2,490	$ 4,339	34	$ 854	$ 2,769	$ 4,532
Medical receptionists	241	$ 11,511	$ 16,617	$ 23,775	47	$ 11,870	$ 18,257	$ 23,047
Medical secretaries, transcribers	210	$ 3,291	$ 6,025	$ 9,689	38	$ 3,376	$ 5,018	$ 10,731
Medical records	215	$ 4,377	$ 6,459	$ 9,596	45	$ 4,383	$ 7,672	$ 11,369
Other administrative support	141	$ 1,212	$ 3,398	$ 8,762	23	$ 836	$ 1,044	$ 4,701
Registered nurses	221	$ 8,699	$ 16,170	$ 28,114	47	$ 8,903	$ 15,691	$ 28,978
Licensed practical nurse	226	$ 6,269	$ 12,189	$ 19,996	39	$ 5,248	$ 10,103	$ 15,702
Medical assistants, nurse aides	228	$ 6,355	$ 11,726	$ 18,319	45	$ 9,702	$ 15,701	$ 22,541
Clinical laboratory	196	$ 5,287	$ 8,681	$ 11,981	43	$ 7,805	$ 9,736	$ 12,833
Radiology and imaging	194	$ 3,417	$ 6,114	$ 11,216	45	$ 5,766	$ 9,003	$ 11,964
Other medical support services	137	$ 3,233	$ 6,727	$ 14,179	35	$ 3,121	$ 6,180	$ 11,758
Total employed support staff cost	280	$ 97,785	$ 124,584	$ 147,356	52	$ 124,712	$ 141,496	$ 175,491
Total employed support staff benefits	272	$ 19,452	$ 27,732	$ 36,692	49	$ 21,694	$ 31,642	$ 42,628
Total contracted support staff	152	$ 2,104	$ 4,291	$ 8,754	34	$ 1,995	$ 5,276	$ 10,110
Total support staff cost	280	$ 120,618	$ 152,853	$ 191,457	52	$ 152,071	$ 181,492	$ 219,584

MGMA Benchmarks—Better Performing Practices Comparison Tables ■ 167

Table 1c. Staff Cost As a Percent of Total Medical Revenue

	Count	Not a Better Performer 25th %tile	Not a Better Performer Median	Not a Better Performer 75th %tile	Count	Better Performer 25th %tile	Better Performer Median	Better Performer 75th %tile
General administrative	246	1.98	2.68	3.87	50	1.73	2.52	3.54
Business office	251	2.65	3.43	4.39	50	2.38	3.09	4.29
Managed care administrative	90	0.25	0.59	1.08	21	0.24	1.01	1.25
Information technology	132	0.39	0.60	0.92	34	0.36	0.53	0.92
Housekeeping, maintenance, security	140	0.20	0.45	0.72	34	0.12	0.44	0.69
Medical receptionists	241	2.06	3.31	5.24	47	1.60	2.71	4.14
Medical secretaries, transcribers	210	0.70	1.26	1.79	38	0.46	0.77	1.56
Medical records	215	0.85	1.26	1.94	45	0.67	1.11	1.54
Other administrative support	141	0.23	0.67	2.03	23	0.12	0.15	1.02
Registered nurses	221	1.73	3.23	5.63	47	1.23	2.03	4.54
Licensed practical nurses	226	1.26	2.46	4.21	39	0.97	1.50	2.31
Medical assistants, nurse aides	228	1.25	2.42	3.68	45	1.54	2.71	3.98
Clinical laboratory	196	1.00	1.64	2.25	43	1.09	1.42	1.79
Radiology and imaging	194	0.75	1.19	1.90	45	0.77	1.40	1.80
Other medical support services	137	0.61	1.24	2.29	35	0.52	0.88	1.63
Total employed support staff cost	280	21.67	25.63	31.03	52	19.85	22.76	26.92
Total employed support staff benefits	272	4.58	5.70	6.94	49	3.82	4.98	6.13
Total contracted support staff	152	0.42	0.90	1.61	34	0.24	0.96	1.43
Total support staff cost	280	27.17	31.86	38.55	52	23.90	28.28	32.93

Table 1d. FTE Staff per FTE Physician (Staff Categories)

	Count	Not a Better Performer 25th %tile	Not a Better Performer Median	Not a Better Performer 75th %tile	Count	Better Performer 25th %tile	Better Performer Median	Better Performer 75th %tile
Administrative and Business Staff per FTE Physician	262	0.76	1.13	1.43	51	1.11	1.38	2.00
Front Office Staff per FTE Physician	262	1.24	1.57	1.91	50	1.36	1.82	2.05
Clinical Staff per FTE Physician	257	1.25	1.49	1.84	49	1.30	1.62	1.95
Ancillary Service Staff per FTE Physician	229	0.33	0.64	0.99	49	0.56	0.81	1.21

Table 1e. Staff Cost per FTE Physician (Staff Categories)

	Count	Not a Better Performer 25th %tile	Not a Better Performer Median	Not a Better Performer 75th %tile	Count	Better Performer 25th %tile	Better Performer Median	Better Performer 75th %tile
Administrative and Business Staff Salary per FTE Physician	262	$ 25,505	$ 34,872	$ 45,175	50	$ 34,167	$ 45,560	$ 58,059
Front Office Staff Salary per FTE Physician	261	$ 24,276	$ 31,267	$ 38,467	49	$ 26,430	$ 35,520	$ 43,011
Clinical Staff Salary per FTE Physician	258	$ 31,248	$ 40,701	$ 51,499	48	$ 33,470	$ 40,594	$ 54,890
Ancillary Service Staff Salary per FTE Physician	231	$ 8,598	$ 18,215	$ 29,073	48	$ 15,540	$ 24,287	$ 35,473

Table 1f. Staff Cost As a Percent of Total Medical Revenue (Staff Categories)

	Count	Not a Better Performer 25th %tile	Not a Better Performer Median	Not a Better Performer 75th %tile	Count	Better Performer 25th %tile	Better Performer Median	Better Performer 75th %tile
Administrative and Business Staff Salary As % of Total Medical Revenue	262	5.43	7.09	8.66	50	5.37	6.92	
Front Office Staff Salary As % of Total Medical Revenue	261	4.76	6.36	8.45	49	3.60	5.64	
Clinical Staff Salary As % of Total Medical Revenue	258	6.42	8.21	11.19	48	5.24	6.82	
Ancillary Service Staff Salary As % of Total Medical Revenue	231	2.16	3.47	4.97	48	2.72	3.86	

168 ■ APPENDIX IV

TABLE 2 ■ Cardiology, Not Hospital/Integrated Delivery System Owned

Table 2a. FTE Staff per FTE Physician

	Count	Not a Better Performer 25th %tile	Median	75th %tile	Count	Better Performer 25th %tile	Median	75th %tile
General administrative	77	0.18	0.25	0.41	15	0.18	0.25	0.35
Business office	76	0.67	0.82	1.00	15	0.63	0.91	1.32
Managed care administrative	21	0.06	0.09	0.14	2	*	*	*
Information technology	31	0.07	0.09	0.14	8	*	*	*
Housekeeping, maintenance, security	5	*	*	*	3	*	*	*
Medical receptionists	77	0.50	0.66	0.94	15	0.36	0.69	1.25
Medical secretaries, transcribers	68	0.25	0.39	0.57	14	0.21	0.25	0.37
Medical records	74	0.25	0.36	0.47	14	0.33	0.41	0.68
Other administrative support	38	0.09	0.16	0.27	9	*	*	*
Registered nurses	74	0.43	0.67	1.16	14	0.36	0.55	0.86
Licensed practical nurses	45	0.10	0.22	0.40	9	*	*	*
Medical assistants, nurse aides	72	0.25	0.50	0.71	15	0.27	0.44	0.88
Clinical laboratory	17	0.08	0.15	0.25	5	*	*	*
Radiology and imaging	64	0.25	0.40	0.63	14	0.25	0.44	0.56
Other medical support services	48	0.23	0.33	0.61	10	0.25	0.65	0.87
Total employed support staff	80	3.68	4.96	6.09	15	3.74	5.09	6.50
Total contracted support staff	43	0.07	0.20	0.42	10	0.17	0.27	0.42
Total support staff	80	3.93	5.03	6.28	15	3.81	5.32	7.00

Table 2b. Staff Cost per FTE Physician

	Count	Not a Better Performer 25th %tile	Median	75th %tile	Count	Better Performer 25th %tile	Median	75th %tile
General administrative	75	$ 13,178	$ 17,000	$ 26,804	15	$ 13,413	$ 17,853	$ 25,953
Business office	74	$ 17,088	$ 22,226	$ 28,295	15	$ 17,102	$ 21,335	$ 45,635
Managed care administrative	20	$ 2,107	$ 3,419	$ 6,459	2	*	*	*
Information technology	31	$ 2,505	$ 3,632	$ 5,365	8	*	*	*
Housekeeping, maintenance, security	5	*	*	*	3	*	*	*
Medical receptionists	75	$ 10,983	$ 15,125	$ 19,917	15	$ 8,754	$ 16,704	$ 25,120
Medical secretaries, transcribers	68	$ 7,265	$ 9,763	$ 14,600	14	$ 5,715	$ 9,688	$ 11,919
Medical records	72	$ 4,608	$ 7,128	$ 10,791	14	$ 5,992	$ 7,257	$ 13,064
Other administrative support	37	$ 1,992	$ 4,667	$ 8,548	8	*	*	*
Registered nurses	72	$ 19,485	$ 27,863	$ 43,909	14	$ 16,665	$ 22,297	$ 35,839
Licensed practical nurses	44	$ 2,682	$ 6,233	$ 12,938	9	*	*	*
Medical assistants, nurse aides	70	$ 6,662	$ 10,851	$ 15,770	15	$ 6,421	$ 9,922	$ 25,297
Clinical laboratory	18	$ 2,585	$ 5,303	$ 7,344	5	*	*	*
Radiology and imaging	62	$ 9,528	$ 16,979	$ 26,776	14	$ 10,895	$ 18,225	$ 24,513
Other medical support services	48	$ 7,136	$ 11,732	$ 22,991	10	$ 8,478	$ 25,780	$ 35,771
Total employed support staff cost	79	$ 119,249	$ 152,746	$ 198,960	15	$ 124,726	$ 174,421	$ 203,699
Total employed support staff benefits	77	$ 30,343	$ 37,485	$ 50,646	15	$ 30,163	$ 36,585	$ 53,011
Total contracted support staff	46	$ 2,722	$ 6,425	$ 11,946	11	$ 963	$ 4,840	$ 12,246
Total support staff cost	80	$ 153,797	$ 193,522	$ 252,523	15	$ 169,906	$ 204,584	$ 248,738

Table 2c. Staff Cost As a Percent of Total Medical Revenue

	Count	Not a Better Performer 25th %tile	Median	75th %tile	Count	Better Performer 25th %tile	Median	75th %tile
General administrative	75	1.55%	2.34%	2.97%	15	1.22%	2.02%	2.54%
Business office	74	2.05%	2.70%	3.33%	15	1.95%	2.29%	3.34%
Managed care administrative	20	0.25%	0.38%	0.75%	2	*	*	*
Information technology	31	0.30%	0.45%	0.59%	8	*	*	*
Housekeeping, maintenance, security	5	*	*	*	3	*	*	*
Medical receptionists	75	1.33%	1.80%	2.35%	15	1.24%	1.72%	2.47%
Medical secretaries, transcribers	68	0.84%	1.19%	1.75%	14	0.61%	0.84%	1.04%
Medical records	72	0.57%	0.86%	1.27%	14	0.52%	0.81%	1.08%
Other administrative support	37	0.22%	0.47%	0.96%	8	*	*	*
Registered nurses	72	2.48%	3.74%	4.83%	14	1.26%	2.34%	3.86%
Licensed practical nurses	44	0.33%	0.65%	1.34%	9	*	*	*
Medical assistants, nurse aides	70	0.67%	1.33%	2.13%	15	0.74%	0.95%	2.05%
Clinical laboratory	18	0.27%	0.59%	0.92%	5	*	*	*
Radiology and imaging	62	1.19%	1.77%	2.73%	14	1.09%	1.70%	2.48%
Other medical support services	48	0.83%	1.61%	2.59%	10	0.79%	2.29%	3.06%
Total employed support staff cost	79	15.66%	18.06%	21.86%	15	13.23%	16.82%	18.83%
Total employed support staff benefits	77	3.62%	4.61%	5.61%	15	2.96%	4.10%	5.20%
Total contracted support staff	46	0.31%	0.83%	1.39%	11	0.11%	0.40%	1.31%
Total support staff cost	80	19.71%	23.75%	28.43%	15	17.31%	20.08%	23.72%

Table 2d. FTE Staff per FTE Physician (Staff Categories)

	Count	Not a Better Performer 25th %tile	Median	75th %tile	Count	Better Performer 25th %tile	Median	75th %tile
Administrative and Business Staff per FTE Physician	78	1.00	1.18	1.47	15	0.91	1.45	2.18
Front Office Staff per FTE Physician	78	1.22	1.51	2.03	15	1.06	1.63	2.19
Clinical Staff per FTE Physician	77	0.95	1.35	1.78	15	1.01	1.17	1.47
Ancillary Service Staff per FTE Physician	73	0.43	0.73	1.00	15	0.54	0.73	1.00

Table 2e. Staff Cost per FTE Physician (Staff Categories)

	Count	Not a Better Performer 25th %tile	Median	75th %tile	Count	Better Performer 25th %tile	Median	75th %tile
Administrative and Business Staff Salary per FTE Physician	76	$33,583	$42,018	$59,770	15	$33,364	$50,582	$77,904
Front Office Staff Salary per FTE Physician	76	$28,395	$36,648	$46,079	15	$25,244	$35,602	$46,621
Clinical Staff Salary per FTE Physician	75	$34,960	$45,522	$61,504	15	$32,286	$35,857	$53,996
Ancillary Service Staff Salary per FTE Physician	71	$18,570	$27,893	$39,887	15	$23,948	$27,248	$40,670

Table 2f. Staff Cost As a Percent of Total Medical Revenue (Staff Categories)

	Count	Not a Better Performer 25th %tile	Median	75th %tile	Count	Better Performer 25th %tile	Median	75th %tile
Administrative and Business Staff Salary As % of Total Medical Revenue	76	4.09%	5.31%	6.38%	15	3.06%	4.96%	6.36%
Front Office Staff Salary As % of Total Medical Revenue	76	3.37%	4.33%	5.28%	15	2.37%	3.30%	4.46%
Clinical Staff Salary As % of Total Medical Revenue	75	4.42%	5.38%	6.84%	15	2.77%	4.23%	5.29%
Ancillary Service Staff Salary As % of Total Medical Revenue	71	2.16%	2.75%	4.41%	15	2.25%	3.05%	3.98%

TABLE 3 ■ Family Practice, Not Hospital/Integrated Delivery System Owned

Table 3a. FTE Staff per FTE Physician

	Count	Not a Better Performer 25th %tile	Median	75th %tile	Count	Better Performer 25th %tile	Median	75th %tile
General administrative	34	0.17	0.24	0.33	15	0.17	0.24	0.32
Business office	38	0.50	0.72	1.11	15	0.67	0.83	1.06
Managed care administrative	11	0.12	0.17	0.25	5	*	*	*
Information technology	5	*	*	*	1	*	*	*
Housekeeping, maintenance, security	11	0.07	0.13	0.33	2	*	*	*
Medical receptionists	37	0.65	1.00	1.25	14	0.75	0.99	1.29
Medical secretaries, transcribers	25	0.17	0.33	0.52	12	0.26	0.38	0.60
Medical records	30	0.28	0.39	0.65	10	0.21	0.50	0.66
Other administrative support	9	*	*	*	4	*	*	*
Registered nurses	32	0.25	0.42	0.77	9	*	*	*
Licensed practical nurses	34	0.24	0.40	0.80	12	0.28	0.39	0.83
Medical assistants, nurse aides	30	0.40	0.74	1.11	14	0.37	0.92	1.09
Clinical laboratory	24	0.18	0.30	0.61	12	0.25	0.37	0.48
Radiology and imaging	18	0.11	0.20	0.34	12	0.16	0.22	0.28
Other medical support services	5	*	*	*	3	*	*	*
Total employed support staff	41	3.98	4.50	5.26	15	4.30	5.04	5.74
Total contracted support staff	10	0.06	0.27	0.44	11	0.11	0.21	0.44
Total support staff	41	4.01	4.50	5.33	15	4.63	5.25	5.96

Table 3b. Staff Cost per FTE Physician

	Count	Not a Better Performer 25th %tile	Median	75th %tile	Count	Better Performer 25th %tile	Median	75th %tile
General administrative	33	$ 8,839	$ 13,750	$ 17,269	15	$ 10,327	$ 12,555	$ 18,599
Business office	38	$ 13,222	$ 18,483	$ 25,464	15	$ 13,356	$ 17,645	$ 24,350
Managed care administrative	11	$ 3,198	$ 4,030	$ 6,194	5	*	*	*
Information technology	5	*	*	*	1	*	*	*
Housekeeping, maintenance, security	11	$ 839	$ 2,184	$ 3,937	2	*	*	*
Medical receptionists	36	$ 12,209	$ 18,844	$ 22,594	14	$ 17,155	$ 19,887	$ 24,354
Medical secretaries, transcribers	25	$ 3,085	$ 7,277	$ 10,026	12	$ 4,220	$ 8,548	$ 11,900
Medical records	29	$ 3,964	$ 5,939	$ 11,588	10	$ 3,758	$ 8,510	$ 12,709
Other administrative support	9	*	*	*	4	*	*	*
Registered nurses	31	$ 7,519	$ 11,886	$ 23,778	9	*	*	*
Licensed practical nurses	32	$ 6,287	$ 10,112	$ 16,908	12	$ 7,034	$ 9,918	$ 18,943
Medical assistants, nurse aides	29	$ 7,350	$ 14,383	$ 24,963	14	$ 6,086	$ 19,754	$ 27,291
Clinical laboratory	23	$ 5,891	$ 9,482	$ 17,035	12	$ 6,894	$ 10,631	$ 12,678
Radiology and imaging	17	$ 3,538	$ 6,799	$ 9,643	12	$ 5,244	$ 7,302	$ 7,868
Other medical support services	6	*	*	*	3	*	*	*
Total employed support staff cost	41	$ 92,483	$ 104,192	$ 130,603	15	$ 109,964	$ 117,467	$ 147,292
Total employed support staff benefits	37	$ 16,318	$ 25,340	$ 35,290	15	$ 20,351	$ 27,768	$ 29,827
Total contracted support staff	11	$ 1,084	$ 2,696	$ 5,801	11	$ 3,522	$ 4,173	$ 10,544
Total support staff cost	41	113,603.82	137,525.00	162,368.67	15	132,100.90	152,812.04	175,926.76

MGMA Benchmarks—Better Performing Practices Comparison Tables ■ 171

Table 3c. Staff Cost As a Percent of Total Medical Revenue

	Count	Not a Better Performer 25th %tile	Median	75th %tile	Count	Better Performer 25th %tile	Median	75th %tile
General administrative	33	2.15%	2.57%	3.73%	15	1.88%	2.32%	4.22%
Business office	38	3.31%	4.35%	5.49%	15	2.73%	3.17%	4.51%
Managed care administrative	11	0.69%	0.89%	1.44%	5	*	*	*
Information technology	5	*	*	*	1	*	*	*
Housekeeping, maintenance, security	11	0.20%	0.55%	0.68%	2	*	*	*
Medical receptionists	36	2.93%	4.39%	5.48%	14	2.98%	4.14%	5.68%
Medical secretaries, transcribers	25	1.05%	1.59%	2.38%	12	0.89%	1.74%	2.10%
Medical records	29	1.21%	1.53%	2.27%	10	0.69%	1.53%	2.43%
Other administrative support	9	*	*	*	4	*	*	*
Registered nurses	31	1.66%	3.30%	4.74%	9	*	*	*
Licensed practical nurses	32	1.42%	2.56%	4.32%	12	1.39%	1.78%	3.00%
Medical assistants, nurse aides	29	1.84%	3.56%	5.39%	14	1.07%	4.39%	5.77%
Clinical laboratory	23	1.35%	2.47%	3.24%	12	1.27%	2.13%	2.80%
Radiology and imaging	17	0.83%	1.20%	1.85%	12	1.02%	1.27%	1.49%
Other medical support services	6	*	*	*	3	*	*	*
Total employed support staff cost	41	23.60%	26.01%	30.83%	15	21.74%	22.34%	29.24%
Total employed support staff benefits	37	4.32%	6.23%	7.36%	15	3.93%	5.31%	6.69%
Total contracted support staff	11	0.27%	0.52%	1.47%	11	0.62%	0.93%	2.01%
Total support staff cost	41	28.59%	32.38%	37.23%	15	26.22%	30.91%	34.08%

Table 3d. FTE Staff per FTE Physician (Staff Categories)

	Count	Not a Better Performer 25th %tile	Median	75th %tile	Count	Better Performer 25th %tile	Median	75th %tile
Administrative and Business Staff per FTE Physician	39	0.80	1.04	1.50	15	0.94	1.21	1.58
Front Office Staff per FTE Physician	38	1.30	1.61	1.95	14	1.50	1.87	2.28
Clinical Staff per FTE Physician	38	1.21	1.49	1.68	15	1.23	1.47	1.88
Ancillary Service Staff per FTE Physician	28	0.25	0.40	0.74	14	0.50	0.56	0.64

Table 3e. Staff Cost per FTE Physician (Staff Categories)

	Count	Not a Better Performer 25th %tile	Median	75th %tile	Count	Better Performer 25th %tile	Median	75th %tile
Administrative and Business Staff Salary per FTE Physician	38	$ 25,560	$ 30,907	$ 42,120	15	$ 28,546	$ 31,995	$ 41,545
Front Office Staff Salary per FTE Physician	37	$ 19,988	$ 28,260	$ 38,330	14	$ 25,442	$ 37,206	$ 48,913
Clinical Staff Salary per FTE Physician	37	$ 29,719	$ 35,788	$ 45,518	15	$ 31,634	$ 35,204	$ 49,605
Ancillary Service Staff Salary per FTE Physician	28	$ 7,361	$ 12,014	$ 19,447	14	$ 12,626	$ 15,819	$ 19,524

Table 3f. Staff Cost As a Percent of Total Medical Revenue (Staff Categories)

	Count	Not a Better Performer 25th %tile	Median	75th %tile	Count	Better Performer 25th %tile	Median	75th %tile
Administrative and Business Staff Salary As % of Total Medical Revenue	38	6.18%	7.13%	9.48%	15	5.15%	6.68%	7.92%
Front Office Staff Salary As % of Total Medical Revenue	37	5.65%	6.64%	9.58%	14	5.38%	7.20%	8.44%
Clinical Staff Salary As % of Total Medical Revenue	37	7.42%	9.01%	10.97%	15	5.81%	7.20%	9.34%
Ancillary Service Staff Salary As % of Total Medical Revenue	28	1.92%	2.87%	5.42%	14	2.47%	2.95%	3.93%

TABLE 4 ■ Obstetrics/Gynecology, Not Hospital/Integrated Delivery System Owned

Table 4a. FTE Staff per FTE Physician

	Count	Not a Better Performer 25th %tile	Median	75th %tile	Count	Better Performer 25th %tile	Median	75th %tile
General administrative	39	0.17	0.20	0.28	9	*	*	*
Business office	40	0.50	0.65	0.81	10	0.63	0.98	1.50
Managed care administrative	4	*	*	*	1	*	*	*
Information technology	4	*	*	*	1	*	*	*
Housekeeping, maintenance, security	1	*	*	*	2	*	*	*
Medical receptionists	39	0.67	0.94	1.12	11	0.78	1.02	1.36
Medical secretaries, transcribers	23	0.10	0.20	0.33	6	*	*	*
Medical records	36	0.18	0.30	0.48	8	*	*	*
Other administrative support	14	0.19	0.45	0.72	5	*	*	*
Registered nurses	33	0.29	0.50	0.88	9	*	*	*
Licensed practical nurses	26	0.23	0.38	0.59	10	0.19	0.33	0.66
Medical assistants, nurse aides	33	0.40	0.83	1.33	11	0.75	1.28	1.69
Clinical laboratory	14	0.15	0.29	0.42	7	*	*	*
Radiology and imaging	24	0.15	0.18	0.25	8	*	*	*
Other medical support services	7	*	*	*	1	*	*	*
Total employed support staff	40	3.48	4.34	5.17	11	4.91	5.83	6.32
Total contracted support staff	21	0.07	0.15	0.21	5	*	*	*
Total support staff	41	3.56	4.29	5.16	11	4.91	5.86	6.39

Table 4b. Staff Cost per FTE Physician

	Count	Not a Better Performer 25th %tile	Median	75th %tile	Count	Better Performer 25th %tile	Median	75th %tile
General administrative	39	$ 10,000	$ 13,378	$ 17,216	9	*	*	*
Business office	39	$ 14,458	$ 17,036	$ 20,240	10	$ 17,513	$ 26,139	$ 36,343
Managed care administrative	5	*	*	*	1	$ 11,980	$ 11,980	$ 11,980
Information technology	5	*	*	*	1	*	*	*
Housekeeping, maintenance, security	1	*	*	*	2	*	*	*
Medical receptionists	38	$ 14,446	$ 19,459	$ 24,287	11	$ 14,237	$ 23,618	$ 28,377
Medical secretaries, transcribers	22	$ 3,019	$ 4,277	$ 8,413	6	*	*	*
Medical records	35	$ 3,355	$ 5,859	$ 9,924	8	*	*	*
Other administrative support	14	$ 4,470	$ 8,964	$ 15,859	5	*	*	*
Registered nurses	32	$ 8,854	$ 17,910	$ 28,664	9	*	*	*
Licensed practical nurses	25	$ 7,661	$ 10,977	$ 16,959	10	$ 5,730	$ 8,704	$ 17,179
Medical assistants, nurse aides	32	$ 10,233	$ 17,831	$ 31,048	11	$ 17,058	$ 29,467	$ 37,926
Clinical laboratory	14	$ 2,833	$ 7,814	$ 15,025	7	*	*	*
Radiology and imaging	23	$ 6,132	$ 9,051	$ 12,218	8	*	*	*
Other medical support services	8	*	*	*	2	*	*	*
Total employed support staff cost	41	$ 98,417	$ 115,211	$ 128,257	11	$ 145,934	$ 161,922	$ 196,608
Total employed support staff benefits	40	$ 23,828	$ 27,776	$ 34,809	11	$ 27,240	$ 31,304	$ 43,336
Total contracted support staff	23	$ 1,262	$ 2,777	$ 5,617	6	*	*	*
Total support staff cost	41	$ 127,138	$ 144,334	$ 167,588	11	$ 176,138	$ 199,319	$ 233,154

MGMA Benchmarks—Better Performing Practices Comparison Tables ■ 173

Table 4c. Staff Cost As a Percent of Total Medical Revenue

	Count	Not a Better Performer 25th %tile	Median	75th %tile	Count	Better Performer 25th %tile	Median	75th %tile
General administrative	39	1.85%	2.54%	2.88%	9	*	*	*
Business office	39	2.52%	3.23%	3.89%	10	2.26%	3.11%	4.52%
Managed care administrative	5	*	*	*	1	*	*	*
Information technology	5	*	*	*	1	*	*	*
Housekeeping, maintenance, security	1	*	*	*	2	*	*	*
Medical receptionists	38	2.72%	3.30%	4.51%	11	1.46%	2.93%	3.58%
Medical secretaries, transcribers	22	0.49%	0.75%	1.62%	6	*	*	*
Medical records	35	0.72%	1.09%	1.62%	8	*	*	*
Other administrative support	14	0.83%	1.36%	2.27%	5	*	*	*
Registered nurses	32	1.61%	3.01%	4.89%	9	*	*	*
Licensed practical nurses	25	1.26%	2.06%	3.05%	10	0.73%	1.12%	1.93%
Medical assistants, nurse aides	32	1.99%	3.42%	4.68%	11	2.20%	3.90%	4.70%
Clinical laboratory	14	0.51%	1.27%	2.66%	7	*	*	*
Radiology and imaging	23	1.01%	1.54%	2.27%	8	*	*	*
Other medical support services	8	*	*	*	2	*	*	*
Total employed support staff cost	41	19.45%	21.03%	22.04%	11	18.50%	21.39%	22.07%
Total employed support staff benefits	40	4.22%	5.09%	6.05%	11	3.25%	4.26%	6.04%
Total contracted support staff	23	0.21%	0.57%	1.11%	6	*	*	*
Total support staff cost	41	24.34%	25.83%	28.07%	11	23.80%	25.76%	27.52%

Table 4d. FTE Staff per FTE Physician (Staff Categories)

	Count	Not a Better Performer 25th %tile	Median	75th %tile	Count	Better Performer 25th %tile	Median	75th %tile
Administrative and Business Staff per FTE Physician	40	0.70	0.92	1.12	10	0.94	1.43	1.83
Front Office Staff per FTE Physician	39	1.10	1.52	1.91	11	1.42	1.54	2.00
Clinical Staff per FTE Physician	40	1.26	1.50	1.83	11	2.22	2.31	2.50
Ancillary Service Staff per FTE Physician	29	0.19	0.29	0.47	9	*	*	*

Table 4e. Staff Cost per FTE Physician (Staff Categories)

	Count	Not a Better Performer 25th %tile	Median	75th %tile	Count	Better Performer 25th %tile	Median	75th %tile
Administrative and Business Staff Salary per FTE Physician	39	$ 25,625	$ 31,165	$ 39,646	10	$ 30,877	$ 47,540	$ 62,910
Front Office Staff Salary per FTE Physician	38	$ 25,636	$ 31,041	$ 40,854	11	$ 31,598	$ 33,913	$ 39,350
Clinical Staff Salary per FTE Physician	39	$ 31,889	$ 40,649	$ 45,995	11	$ 55,405	$ 64,041	$ 79,884
Ancillary Service Staff Salary per FTE Physician	28	$ 7,907	$ 11,512	$ 16,784	9	*	*	*

Table 4f. Staff Cost As a Percent of Total Medical Revenue (Staff Categories)

	Count	Not a Better Performer 25th %tile	Median	75th %tile	Count	Better Performer 25th %tile	Median	75th %tile
Administrative and Business Staff Salary As % of Total Medical Revenue	39	4.72%	5.87%	6.98%	10	3.91%	6.29%	7.67%
Front Office Staff Salary As % of Total Medical Revenue	38	4.42%	5.77%	7.29%	11	3.58%	4.24%	5.20%
Clinical Staff Salary As % of Total Medical Revenue	39	6.12%	7.15%	8.50%	11	7.15%	8.04%	9.55%
Ancillary Service Staff Salary As % of Total Medical Revenue	28	1.35%	1.85%	3.18%	9	*	*	*

174 ■ APPENDIX IV

TABLE 5 ■ Orthopedic Surgery, Not Hospital/Integrated Delivery System Owned

Table 5a. FTE Staff per FTE Physician

	\multicolumn{4}{c}{Not a Better Performer}		\multicolumn{4}{c}{Better Performer}
	Count	25th %tile	Median	75th %tile	Count	25th %tile	Median	75th %tile
General administrative	89	0.17	0.25	0.35	27	0.17	0.30	0.40
Business office	90	0.63	0.85	1.22	28	0.87	1.13	1.39
Managed care administrative	19	0.08	0.14	0.23	6	*	*	*
Information technology	39	0.07	0.11	0.23	9	*	*	*
Housekeeping, maintenance, security	21	0.04	0.12	0.23	3	*	*	*
Medical receptionists	90	0.66	0.85	1.04	27	0.79	1.21	1.43
Medical secretaries, transcribers	82	0.31	0.49	0.88	24	0.42	0.74	1.12
Medical records	78	0.21	0.32	0.50	26	0.31	0.44	0.61
Other administrative support	40	0.07	0.15	0.58	7	*	*	*
Registered nurses	57	0.16	0.30	0.70	15	0.15	0.17	0.33
Licensed practical nurses	40	0.11	0.25	0.48	7	*	*	*
Medical assistants, nurse aides	75	0.26	0.56	0.91	23	0.49	0.88	1.19
Clinical laboratory	6	*	*	*	3	*	*	*
Radiology and imaging	85	0.34	0.45	0.58	27	0.37	0.50	0.69
Other medical support services	41	0.24	0.38	0.82	13	0.21	0.50	0.83
Total employed support staff	94	3.81	4.75	5.71	28	4.69	5.67	6.58
Total contracted support staff	38	0.09	0.20	0.31	11	0.14	0.23	0.45
Total support staff	94	3.82	4.87	5.83	28	4.90	6.01	6.69

Table 5b. Staff Cost per FTE Physician

	\multicolumn{4}{c}{Not a Better Performer}		\multicolumn{4}{c}{Better Performer}
	Count	25th %tile	Median	75th %tile	Count	25th %tile	Median	75th %tile
General administrative	87	$ 11,480	$ 17,236	$ 20,741	27	$ 15,497	$ 18,019	$ 24,483
Business office	88	$ 17,760	$ 23,108	$ 29,954	28	$ 23,964	$ 30,022	$ 38,367
Managed care administrative	19	$ 2,250	$ 4,142	$ 7,578	6	*	*	*
Information technology	40	$ 2,469	$ 3,991	$ 6,391	9	*	*	*
Housekeeping, maintenance, security	24	$ 550	$ 2,706	$ 3,977	3	*	*	*
Medical receptionists	87	$ 13,283	$ 18,837	$ 24,930	27	$ 16,965	$ 25,496	$ 40,416
Medical secretaries, transcribers	79	$ 8,101	$ 13,189	$ 21,294	23	$ 10,899	$ 24,618	$ 32,290
Medical records	75	$ 4,212	$ 6,533	$ 10,009	26	$ 6,166	$ 7,270	$ 12,185
Other administrative support	38	$ 1,442	$ 4,081	$ 12,191	7	*	*	*
Registered nurses	56	$ 7,835	$ 13,058	$ 25,626	15	$ 5,716	$ 7,833	$ 13,799
Licensed practical nurses	38	$ 3,911	$ 7,123	$ 16,056	7	*	*	*
Medical assistants, nurse aides	71	$ 7,614	$ 14,878	$ 25,740	23	$ 13,523	$ 31,135	$ 37,624
Clinical laboratory	6	*	*	*	3	*	*	*
Radiology and imaging	82	$ 11,586	$ 14,650	$ 17,580	27	$ 12,451	$ 16,526	$ 22,672
Other medical support services	40	$ 7,319	$ 12,072	$ 31,432	13	$ 7,005	$ 18,444	$ 25,087
Total employed support staff cost	93	$ 111,997	$ 137,956	$ 171,529	28	$ 138,645	$ 172,935	$ 194,087
Total employed support staff benefits	88	$ 25,520	$ 32,651	$ 46,165	28	$ 33,508	$ 40,597	$ 46,743
Total contracted support staff	44	$ 2,136	$ 7,044	$ 12,328	14	$ 2,284	$ 5,387	$ 11,996
Total support staff cost	94	$ 140,654	$ 173,409	$ 218,741	28	$ 176,817	$ 215,464	$ 240,204

MGMA Benchmarks—Better Performing Practices Comparison Tables ■ 175

Table 5c. Staff Cost As a Percent of Total Medical Revenue

		Not a Better Performer				Better Performer		
	Count	25th %tile	Median	75th %tile	Count	25th %tile	Median	75th %tile
General administrative	87	1.56%	2.30%	2.82%	27	1.65%	1.95%	2.54%
Business office	88	2.24%	3.19%	4.07%	28	2.51%	3.18%	3.80%
Managed care administrative	19	0.32%	0.54%	0.95%	6	*	*	*
Information technology	40	0.30%	0.57%	0.77%	9	*	*	*
Housekeeping, maintenance, security	24	0.07%	0.30%	0.48%	3	*	*	*
Medical receptionists	87	1.56%	2.48%	3.58%	27	2.04%	2.93%	3.84%
Medical secretaries, transcribers	79	1.12%	1.74%	3.08%	23	1.17%	2.71%	3.64%
Medical records	75	0.54%	0.81%	1.17%	26	0.58%	0.89%	1.25%
Other administrative support	38	0.19%	0.49%	1.77%	7	*	*	*
Registered nurses	56	0.97%	1.93%	3.22%	15	0.53%	0.85%	1.27%
Licensed practical nurses	38	0.46%	0.98%	2.00%	7	*	*	*
Medical assistants, nurse aides	71	0.96%	1.80%	3.23%	23	1.42%	3.09%	3.96%
Clinical laboratory	6	*	*	*	3	*	*	*
Radiology and imaging	82	1.42%	1.83%	2.57%	27	1.18%	1.70%	2.24%
Other medical support services	40	0.98%	1.64%	3.32%	13	0.67%	1.22%	2.71%
Total employed support staff cost	93	15.40%	18.34%	21.03%	28	14.48%	18.19%	21.22%
Total employed support staff benefits	88	3.54%	4.37%	5.51%	28	3.20%	4.36%	5.17%
Total contracted support staff	44	0.24%	1.02%	1.86%	14	0.21%	0.62%	1.40%
Total support staff cost	94	20.50%	23.58%	26.52%	28	20.30%	22.10%	26.40%

Table 5d. FTE Staff per FTE Physician (Staff Categories)

		Not a Better Performer				Better Performer		
	Count	25th %tile	Median	75th %tile	Count	25th %tile	Median	75th %tile
Administrative and Business Staff per FTE Physician	93	0.98	1.26	1.63	28	1.18	1.39	1.94
Front Office Staff per FTE Physician	92	1.37	1.81	2.31	28	2.05	2.47	2.83
Clinical Staff per FTE Physician	87	0.66	1.00	1.38	26	0.69	1.12	1.34
Ancillary Service Staff per FTE Physician	89	0.43	0.59	0.89	27	0.50	0.69	0.98

Table 5e. Staff Cost per FTE Physician (Staff Categories)

		Not a Better Performer				Better Performer		
	Count	25th %tile	Median	75th %tile	Count	25th %tile	Median	75th %tile
Administrative and Business Staff Salary per FTE Physician	91	$ 33,082	$ 42,623	$ 56,259	28	$ 43,821	$ 48,815	$ 67,025
Front Office Staff Salary per FTE Physician	89	$ 32,510	$ 42,097	$ 53,558	28	$ 40,149	$ 61,511	$ 74,613
Clinical Staff Salary per FTE Physician	84	$ 18,900	$ 28,624	$ 44,959	26	$ 23,299	$ 33,022	$ 45,837
Ancillary Service Staff Salary per FTE Physician	86	$ 13,319	$ 19,388	$ 29,359	27	$ 16,237	$ 21,272	$ 30,899

Table 5f. Staff Cost As a Percent of Total Medical Revenue (Staff Categories)

		Not a Better Performer				Better Performer		
	Count	25th %tile	Median	75th %tile	Count	25th %tile	Median	75th %tile
Administrative and Business Staff Salary As % of Total Medical Revenue	91	4.46%	5.97%	7.26%	28	4.38%	5.36%	6.86%
Front Office Staff Salary As % of Total Medical Revenue	89	4.48%	5.58%	7.27%	28	4.80%	6.81%	7.93%
Clinical Staff Salary As % of Total Medical Revenue	84	2.60%	3.73%	5.20%	26	2.05%	3.73%	4.40%
Ancillary Service Staff Salary As % of Total Medical Revenue	86	1.88%	2.59%	3.89%	27	1.78%	2.23%	3.25%

Appendix V
MGMA Definitions of Support Staff Positions

This appendix contains definitions for support staff positions based on definitions used in the MGMA Cost Survey report. To compute the full-time-equivalency (FTE) of the practice's employees, add the number of full-time (1.0 FTE) support staff to the FTE count for the part-time support staff. A full-time employee works the number of hours the practice considers to be a normal workweek. In most medical practices this is 37.5 hours (five 7.5-hour workdays per week) or 40 hours (five 8.0-hour workdays per week). To compute the FTE of a part-time support staff employee, divide the total hours worked in an average week by the number of hours that your practice considers to be a normal workweek. For example, an employee working 30 hours in a practice with a normal workweek of 40 hours would be 0.75 FTE (30 divided by 40 hours). Note, an employee should not be counted as more than 1.0 FTE, regardless of the number of hours worked.

Medical practice staff members can be grouped into four major classifications:

1. Administrative and Business Staff
2. Front Office Staff
3. Clinical Staff
4. Ancillary Service Staff

Each major classification can be further segmented by the specific position of the staff member.

The following are the general guidelines for classifying staff members.

1. Administrative and Business Staff consist of staff members supporting the general administration of the practice, including:

General administrative: The general administrative and practice management staff and supporting secretaries, administrative assistants, etc. including: executive staff, such as administrator, assistant administrator, chief financial officer, medical director, other directors (such as director of nursing), site managers, human resources staff, marketing staff and purchasing department staff. Do not include: directors of support or ancillary departments, such as the laboratory director, radiology director, or information technology director that are reported in their respective areas.

Business office: The business office staff, such as business office manager, secretaries and the insurance, billing, credit, accounting, cashiering, collections, bookkeeping, charge entry and accounting data input staff.

Managed care administrative: The managed care administrative staff and supporting secretaries, administrative assistants, including HMO/PPO contract administrators, case management staff, actuaries, managed care medical directors and managed care marketing, quality assurance and utilization review staff.

Information technology: The data processing, computer programming and telecommunications staff.

Housekeeping, maintenance, security: The housekeeping, maintenance and security staff for the practice.

2. Front Office Staff consist of staff members in the following functions:

Medical receptionists: The medical receptionists, switchboard operators, schedulers and appointment staff.

Medical secretaries, transcribers: medical secretaries, transcribers and clerks.

Medical records: medical records, coding staff and X-ray film library staff.

Other administrative support: other administrative staff such as mail room, cafeteria and laundry staff.

3. Clinical Staff consist of employees who assist physicians in patient care in the following functions:

Registered Nurses: Registered nurse staff and registered nurses working as frontline managers or lead nurses. Do not include midlevel providers such as nurse practitioners, Certified Registered Nurse Anesthetists (CRNA), or nurse midwives.

Licensed Practical Nurses: Licensed practical nurses and licensed vocational nurses and equivalent nursing staff with state licenses.

Medical assistants, nurse's aides: medical assistants and nurse's aides.

4. Ancillary Service Staff consist of employees who are directly associated with the following services:

Clinical laboratory: The clinical laboratory and pathology department conducts procedures for clinical laboratory and pathology CPT codes 80048-89399.

Radiology and imaging: The diagnostic radiology and imaging department conducts procedures for diagnostic radiology CPT codes 70010-76499, diagnostic ultrasound CPT codes 76506-76999 and diagnostic nuclear medicine CPT codes 78000-78999.

Other medical support services: FTE and cost of support staff in other ancillary services departments, such as physical therapy, optical, ambulatory surgery, electrocardiograph, radiation oncology, therapeutic nuclear medicine, etc.

Total Contracted Support Staff

In addition to the four major staff classifications, some medical practices have engaged contracted support services. Contracted support staff represents individuals hired on a contract or temporary basis that are not employed by the medical practice.

Source: Cost Survey: 2001 Report Based on 2000 Data. Englewood, CO: Medical Group Management Association, 2001.